INTRACARDIAC ECHOCARDIOGRAPHY IN INTERVENTIONAL ELECTROPHYSIOLOGY

INTRACARDIAC ECHOCARDIOGRAPHY IN INTERVENTIONAL ELECTROPHYSIOLOGY

Editor

Andrea Natale MD
Department of Cardiology
Cleveland Clinic Foundation
Cleveland, OH
USA

Co-editors

David J Wilber MD
Cardiovascular Institute
Loyola University Medical Center
Maywood, IL
USA

John F Rhodes Jr MD
Division of Pediatric Cardiology
Duke University Medical Center
Durham, NC
USA

Vivek Reddy MD
Cardiac Unit Associates
Massachusetts General Hospital
Boston, MA
USA

Antonio Raviele MD
Division of Cardiology
Umberto I Hospital
Mestre-Venice
Italy

Luc Jordaens MD PhD
Department of Cardiology
Erasmus Medical Centre
Rotterdam
The Netherlands

Jonathan M Kalman MBBS PhD FRACP
Department of Cardiology
Royal Melbourne Hospital
Melbourne, VIC
Australia

informa
healthcare

New York London

First published in 2006 by the Taylor & Francis Group.

This edition published in 2010 by Informa Healthcare, Telephone House, 69-77 Paul Street, London EC2A 4LQ, UK.

Simultaneously published in the USA by Informa Healthcare, 52 Vanderbilt Avenue, 7th Floor, New York, NY 10017, USA.

Informa Healthcare is a trading division of Informa UK Ltd. Registered Office: 37–41 Mortimer Street, London W1T 3JH, UK. Registered in England and Wales number 1072954.

A CIP record for this book is available from the British Library.

Library of Congress Cataloging-in-Publication Data available on application

ISBN-13: 9781842143100

Orders may be sent to: Informa Healthcare, Sheepen Place, Colchester, Essex CO3 3LP, UK
Telephone: +44 (0)20 7017 5540
Email: CSDhealthcarebooks@informa.com
Website: http://informahealthcarebooks.com/

For corporate sales please contact: CorporateBooksIHC@informa.com
For foreign rights please contact: RightsIHC@informa.com
For reprint permissions please contact: PermissionsIHC@informa.com

Contents

Acknowledgments   vii

List of Contributors   ix

1   Introduction   1
    Dimpi Patel, Hanka Mlcochova, David Burkhardt, and James Thomas

2   Atrial chambers: gross anatomy and intracardiac phased-array echocardiography imaging   11
    Sakis Themistoclakis, Aldo Bonso, Antonio Rossillo, and Antonio Raviele

3   The interatrial septum   31
    Samir Kapadia, Atul Verma, Oussama Wazni, and Leonardo Rodriguez

4   Role of intracardiac echocardiography for ablation of ventricular tachycardia   39
    David J Wilber and Neil Brysiewicz

5   Abnormal anatomy: left atrial structures   45
    Omosalewa O Lalude and Allan L Klein

6   Intracardiac echocardiography during catheter ablation for atrial fibrillation   59
    Mandeep Bhargava, Robert A Schweikert, Steven Hao, and Andrea Natale

7   Transcatheter occlusion of left atrial appendage for stroke prevention in
    atrial fibrillation – potential role for intracardiac echocardiography   91
    *Hsuan-Hung Chuang, Dhanunjaya Lakkireddy, Jennifer Cummings, and
    E Murat Tuzcu*

8   Intracardiac echocardiography: transseptal catheterization   99
    Walid Saliba, Jennifer E Cummings, Gery Tomassoni, and Andrea Natale

9   Right atrium: ICE in anatomic definition, mapping and ablation   105
    Richard J Hillock, Joseph B Morton, and Jonathan M Kalman

10 Intracardiac echocardiography in the congenital catheterization laboratory   115
    Piers CA Barker and John F Rhodes Jr

11 Intrapericardial echocardiography: a novel catheter-based approach to
    cardiac imaging   129
    Ana Clara Tude Rodrigues, Andre d'Avila, Vivek Y Reddy, and Eduardo Saad

12 Three-dimensional echocardiography – future applications in interventional cardiology   133
    Hsuan-Hung Chuang, Tamas Szili-Torok, Luc J Jordaens, and Takahiro Shiota

13 The future of image-guided therapies in interventional electrophysiology   145
    Dimpi Patel, Marcoen F Scholten, Robert Savage, and Vivek Y Reddy

Index   153

Dedication

To my wife, Marina, for her endless love, understanding and faith in me, and to my daughters in the hope to teach them that whatever they do in life to do it with passion

Acknowledgments

Our deep appreciation and thanks to Dr Dimpi Patel, who coordinated the efforts of all our contributing authors. With her patience and grace, she has managed to keep all of us on track and facilitated our communications. We also gratefully acknowledge the invaluable assistance and support of our AF nurses; Michelle Williams-Andrews, Minerva Sherman, Christina Magnelli-Reyes, Jocelyn Butler, Stacy Poe, Sue Sima, Lisa Keene, Charlene Bielik, and Barbara Thomas, a most effective team without whose support we would be lost. Day after day, they are of enormous help in their countless efforts and they provide our patients with world class care.

We cannot thank enough our many contributors and colleagues who labored extensively, often taking time away from their families and professional duties, to finish their chapters.

Our hope is that this book will be a valuable tool and reference for clinicians and will help them to make decisions that improve their patients' lives.

Contributors

Piers CA Barker MD
Division of Pediatric Cardiology
Duke University Medical Center
Durham, NC
USA

Mandeep Bhargava MD
Section of Pacing and Electrophysiology
The Cleveland Clinic Foundation
Cleveland, OH
USA

Aldo Bonso MD
Cardiology Unit
Cardiovascular Department
Umberto I Hospital
Mestre-Venice
Italy

Neil Brysiewicz BSE
Cardiovascular Institute
Loyola University Medical Center
Maywood, IL
USA

J David Burkhardt MD
Section of Pacing and Electrophysiology
The Cleveland Clinic Foundation
Cleveland, OH
USA

Hsuan-Hung Chuang MD MBBS MRCP(UK) MED-FAMS
Section of Cardiovascular Imaging
The Cleveland Clinic Foundation
Cleveland, OH
USA

Jennifer E Cummings MD
Section of Pacing and Electrophysiology
The Cleveland Clinic Foundation
Cleveland, OH
USA

Andre d'Avila MD PhD
Cardiac Arrhythmia and Pacemaker Unit
Hospital Pró-Cardíaco
Rio de Janeiro
Brazil

Steven Hao MD
California Pacific Medical Center
San Francisco, CA
USA

Richard J Hillock MBChB FRACP
Department of Cardiology
Christchurch Hospital
New Zealand

Luc J Jordaens MD PhD
Department of Cardiology
Erasmus Medical Center
Rotterdam
The Netherlands

Jonathan M Kalman MBBS FRACP PhD
Department of Cardiology
Royal Melbourne Hospital
Melbourne, VIC
Australia

Samir Kapadia MD
Section of Interventional Cardiology
The Cleveland Clinic Foundation
Cleveland, OH
USA

Allan L Klein MD FRCP(C) FACC
Director of Cardiovascular Imaging Research
Section of Cardiovascular Imaging
The Cleveland Clinic Foundation
Cleveland, OH
USA

Dhanunjaya Lakkireddy MD
Section of Pacing and Electrophysiology
The Cleveland Clinic Foundation
Cleveland, OH
USA

Omosalewa O Lalude MBBS
Section of Cardiovascular Imaging
The Cleveland Clinic Foundation
Cleveland, OH
USA

Hanka Mlcochova MD
Department of Electrophysiology
Institut Klinicke a Experimentalni Mediciny
Prague
Czech Republic

Joseph B Morton MBBS FRACP PhD
Department of Cardiology
Royal Melbourne Hospital
Melbourne, VIC
Australia

Andrea Natale MD
Co-section Head of Section of Pacing and
    Electrophysiology and Director of the
    Electrophysiology Laboratories, and Medical
    Director of the Atrial Fibrillation Center
The Cleveland Clinic Foundation
Cleveland, OH
USA

Dimpi Patel DO
Section of Pacing and Electrophysiology
The Cleveland Clinic Foundation
Cleveland, OH
USA

Antonio Raviele MD
Cardiology Unit
Cardiovascular Department
Umberto I Hospital
Mestre-Venice
Italy

Vivek Y Reddy MD
Massachusetts General Hospital
Cardiac Unit Associates
Boston, MA
USA

John F Rhodes Jr MD
Division of Pediatric Cardiology
Duke University Medical Center
Durham, NC
USA

Ana Clara Tude Rodrigues MD PhD
Echocardiography Laboratory and Cardiology
    Division
Heart Institute
University of São Paulo Medical School
São Paulo, Brasil

Leonardo Rodriguez MD
Section of Cardiovascular Imaging
The Cleveland Clinic Foundation
Cleveland, OH, USA

Antonio Rossillo MD
Cardiology Unit
Cardiovascular Department
Umberto I Hospital
Mestre-Venice
Italy

Eduardo Saad MD
Cardiac Arrhythmia and Pacemaker Unit
Hospital Pró-Cardíaco
Rio de Janeiro
Brazil

Walid Saliba MD
Section of Pacing and Electrophysiology
The Cleveland Clinic Foundation
Cleveland, OH
USA

Robert Savage MD
Section of Cardiothoracic Anesthesiology
The Cleveland Clinic Foundation
Cleveland, OH
USA

Marcoen F Scholten MD
Department of Cardiology
Erasmus Medical Center
Rotterdam
The Netherlands

Robert A Schweikert MD
Section of Pacing and Electrophysiology
The Cleveland Clinic Foundation
Cleveland, OH
USA

Takahiro Shiota MD FACC
Section of Cardiovascular Imaging
The Cleveland Clinic Foundation
Cleveland, OH
USA

Tamas Szili-Torok MD
Department of Cardiology
Erasmus Medical Center
Rotterdam
The Netherlands

Sakis Themistoclakis MD
Cardiology Unit
Cardiovascular Department
Umberto I Hospital
Mestre-Venice
Italy

James Thomas MD
Section Head of Cardiovascular Imaging
The Cleveland Clinic Foundation
Cleveland, OH
USA

Gery Tomassoni MD
Director of the Section of Pacing and Electrophysiology
Central Baptist Hospital
Lexington, KY
USA

E Murat Tuzcu MD
Section of Interventional Cardiology
The Cleveland Clinic Foundation
Cleveland, OH
USA

Atul Verma MD
Section of Pacing and Electrophysiology
The Cleveland Clinic Foundation
Cleveland, OH
USA

Oussama Wazni MD
Section of Pacing and Electrophysiology
The Cleveland Clinic Foundation
Cleveland, OH
USA

David J Wilber MD
Cardiovascular Institute
Loyola University Medical Center
Maywood, IL
USA

Chapter 1 Introduction

Dimpi Patel, Hanka Mlcochova, David Burkhardt, and James Thomas

INTRODUCTION

In 1880 Pierre Curie introduced simple echo sounding methods, which led to the discovery of sonar. Developed during World War I for the navigation of submarines, sonar was shrouded in secrecy until the end of World War II, when it became available to nongovernment scientists to explore its other potential uses. In the early 1950s Edler and Hertz first applied ultrasound imaging to the heart, with the initial application of distinguishing mitral regurgitation from stenosis. A catheter-based ultrasound imaging system was first described by Ciezynski in 1960.[1] Since then, a large array of catheter-based ultrasound imaging systems have been developed and used in clinical practice. In the 1970s and 1980s ultrasound became a formidable medical diagnostic tool in the field of cardiology, particularly with the perfection of pulsed-wave, continuous-wave, and color flow Doppler. Imaging has become essential in assessing cardiac anatomy, function, perfusion, and metabolism. These revolutionary advances seen over the past 20 years occurred primarily because of improvements in computer technology and digital signal processing.

Historically, electrophysiologists have predominantly used fluoroscopy as the primary imaging tool during interventional procedures.[1] However, fluoroscopy, though providing a good two-dimensional (2D) representation of cardiac anatomy, requires significant experience to accurately position interventional devices at an exact intracardiac site.[1-3] Furthermore, fluoroscopy is unable to identify some key anatomic locations (e.g. crista terminalis, coronary sinus (CS) os, superior vena cava (SVC), inferior vena cava (IVC), pulmonary veins (PVs), fossa ovalis, atrial/ventricular relationships to valves, the infarct border zone), to monitor catheter contact, to assess lesion creation, and to visualize extracardiac structures. The recent and rapid development of percutaneous interventional techniques necessitated the development of other technologies.[1,2] Transesophageal echocardiography (TEE) provides excellent visualization of endocardial, epicardial, and valvular structures, but this modality is limited owing to patient discomfort and the need for airway management during prolonged procedures, and the necessity for a second cardiologist.[1-3] These drawbacks created an impetus for researchers to find an alternative imaging modality. Intracardiac echocardiography (ICE) was able to provide accurate images without airway intrusion and has now become the preferred method of imaging.

The two most commonly used ICE systems are mechanical/rotational and phased-array transducers. Mechanical transducers are driven at frequencies of 9 MHz or higher. They have a rotating single piezoelectric element transducer (1800 rpm) which is able to create a circular scan path that is perpendicular to the long axis of a 6F–10F catheter.[1-4] They are able to provide a radial cross-sectional image (10° oblique) and a 10 cm radial imaging depth, with approximately 0.2 mm resolution (Figure 1.1). The miniaturization of these piezoelectric elements was necessary in order to have smaller, more viable catheters. However, the reduced size of the piezoelectric crystals requires transducers to be driven at higher frequencies (10–20 MHz), thus inherently limiting the depth of ultrasound penetration into the tissue. Although mechanical rotational catheters are able to produce high-quality images at shallow depths, they are limited by their stiffness as a result of their rotational core.[1,2,4] Mechanical transducers have been used to visualize the membranous fossa ovalis, crista terminalis, tricuspid annulus, SVC and many other cardiac structures.[1-3] Although this technology has been used occasionally in electrophysiology to visualize the right atrium, mechanical transducers have experienced the greatest success in assessing coronary artery stenosis and guiding stent deployment and placement.[1,2] In contrast, the electrophysiology world has largely

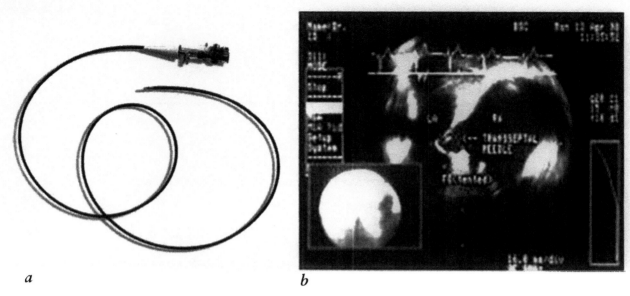

a   *b*

Figure 1.1   *(a) Mechanical/rotational ICE catheters (Boston Scientific) are used at frequencies of 9 MHz or higher. They have a rotating single piezoelectric transducer which is able to create a circular scan path that is perpendicular to the long axis of a 9F catheter. (b) Image attained by a mechanical/rotational catheter visualizing a transseptal needle "tenting" the interatrial septum.*

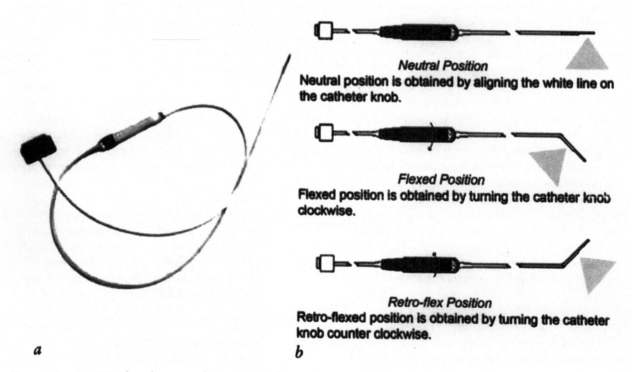

a   *b*

Figure 1.2   *(a) ICE phased-array catheters (EP Medsystems) use a 64 piezoelectric element linear array transducer which operates at a frequency of 7.5 MHz to produce a linear-arc scan path that is perpendicular to the long axis of a 10F catheter. (b) A schematic drawing illustrating the different positions of articulation.*

embraced an ICE phased-array system that uses a 64 piezoelectric element linear array transducer operating at frequencies of 5.5, 7.5, 8.5, and 10 MHz to produce a sector scan parallel to the long axis of a 10F (3.2 mm) catheter[1,2,4] (Figure 1.2).

Another single plane phased-array system produces a linear-arc parallel to the long axis of a 10F catheter and is driven at a frequency of 7.5 MHz (Figure 1.3). The ICE phased-array system is a miniaturized low-frequency transducer that is capable of producing high-resolution, detailed 2D ultrasound images with tissue penetration ranging from 2 mm to 12 cm. Although it images only in a single linear plane, the catheter tip is capable of four-way articulation, thus providing images at multiple angles.[1,2] ICE has gained acceptance as a useful tool in interventional electrophysiology procedures. In this chapter, we will cover the basics of sonography, the indications and contraindications of ICE use, and the rationale for implementing ICE in interventional electrophysiology.

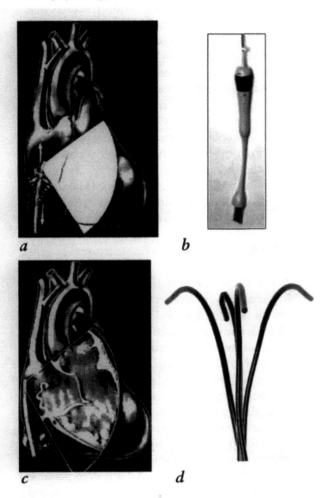

Figure 1.3 *(a) ICE phased-array catheters (Acuson) use a 64 piezoelectric element linear array transducer which operates at frequencies of 5.5–10 MHz to produce a sector scan path that is perpendicular to the long axis of a 10F or 8F catheter. On the handle is a dial that allows the operator to move anterior/posterior/right/left. This deflectable catheter is also able to provide Doppler and color flow imaging. (b,c) A drawing of the ICE catheter illustrating the 90°-shaped sector scan path and the articulation of the catheter within the heart. (d) Although the catheter is only able to image in a single plane, the catheter tip is able to articulate in four directions. With thanks to Starr Kaplan MD for 1.3a and c.*

THE BASICS OF SONOGRAPHY

Piezoelectric crystal transducers are needed to generate ultrasound waves and receive the returning echoes. Molecular dipoles within these ceramic crystals distort the surface when a high voltage is applied, producing vibrations that propagate outward as sound waves, which propagate through the body as a longitudinal traveling wave, displacing the tissue back and forth by a microscopic amount parallel to the sound propagation (Figure 1.4). The process reverses itself when sound strikes the crystal surface, vibrating the molecular dipoles and producing a miniscule electrical signal that can be amplified and displayed as an image.

The journey of an ultrasound wave through human tissue is complex. As waves propagate through different biologic media, they are subject to reflection, refraction, scattering, and absorption (Figure 1.5). Ultrasound waves generally decrease exponentially in amplitude as they pass through homogeneous tissue, with an attenuation coefficient that is specific to the tissue and increasing at higher frequencies, thus limiting the frequency that can be used clinically with echocardiography (Figure 1.6). Whenever an ultrasonic wave encounters a boundary between two tissues the energy is partially reflected, with the remainder being transmitted into the second tissue. The proportion of energy that is transmitted is determined by the difference in acoustic impedances (Z) of the two tissues. Acoustic impedance is defined as the product of sound velocity c and tissue density ρ:

$$Z = \rho c$$

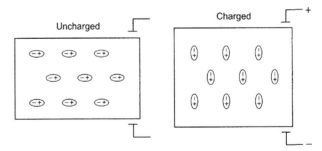

Figure 1.4 *When a voltage is applied across the surface of the piezoelectric crystal, the highly polarized ovoid structures rotate, causing the crystal to thicken and produce ultrasound. When an ultrasound wave is received, the mechanical vibrations of these structures generate an electrical field. (Adapted from Fozzard HA et al (eds), The Heart and Cardiovascular System, 2nd edn. New York: Raven, 1992:635, and from Topol EJ (ed.), Textbook of Cardiovascular Medicine, 2nd edn. Philadelphia: Lippincott, Williams and Wilkins, 2002:CD 46.4.1, with permission.)*

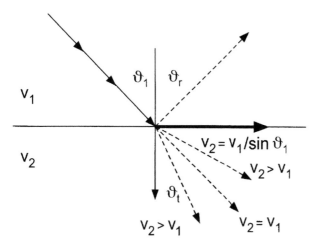

Figure 1.5 *Snell's law. Ultrasound is reflected at the angle of incidence* ($\theta_r = \theta_i$). *The transmitted wave is bent to an angle* θ_t, *such that* $\sin \theta_t = (v_2/v_1) \sin \theta_1$. *If* $(v_2/v_1) \sin \theta_1$ *is greater than 1, then no transmission can occur. (Adapted from Fozzard HA et al (eds), The Heart and Cardiovascular System, 2nd edn. New York: Raven, 1992:636, and from Topol EJ (ed.), Textbook of Cardiovascular Medicine, 2nd edn. Philadelphia: Lippincott, Williams and Wilkins, 2002:CD 46.4.2, with permission.)*

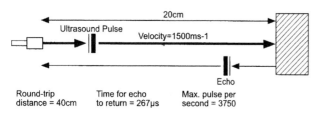

- For depth d, time t, and speed of sound c (1500 – 1540 m/sec):
- $d = ct/2 \approx 77t$ (d in cm, t in ms)
- Maximal pulse repetition frequency: PRF = $c/2d \approx 77/d$

Figure 1.6 *Basics of echocardiographic imaging. Sound propagates through tissue at a relatively fixed speed; therefore, the delay in echo return can be translated into the distance to the reflection. (Adapted from Topol EJ (ed.), Textbook of Cardiovascular Medicine, 2nd edn. Philadelphia: Lippincott, Williams and Wilkins, 2002:CD 46.5, with permission.)*

For large (relative to a wavelength of sound), flat boundaries, the amount of reflected (I_r) energy is given by:

$$I_r = I_i[Z_2 - Z_1]/(Z_2 + Z_1)]^2$$

where I_i is the incident intensity and Z_1 and Z_2 are the impedances for the two tissues. A large difference in impedance between two tissue boundaries results in more energy being reflected than in those

tissue boundaries where the acoustic properties are similar. For instance, the heart–lung interface reflects 54% of the incident ultrasound waves, whereas the blood–myocardium boundary reflects less than 0.1%. As the portion of the wave that was not reflected passes into the next layer of tissue, it will be refracted, thus traveling in a different direction if the velocity of sound differs in the two media. This is generally not a major concern in echocardiography, because the sound velocity between blood and tissue is not great.

When ultrasound waves interact with structures that are smaller than the wavelength of sound, scattering occurs and the small object radiates sound outward as 3D spherical waves. Scattering intensity varies approximately with the sixth power of the particle radius and the fourth power of the ultrasound frequency. Scattering occurs within the tissue at inhomogeneities between cellular and matrix elements that are not simple point scatters. Furthermore, these structures are so close to each other that the reflected waves interfere with each other, producing a complex ultrasound pattern, termed speckle. Thus, in echocardiography, short pulses of ultrasound are scattered, attenuated, and refracted as they propagate from each tissue boundary to the next with a small amount of energy being reflected from the deep structures to the transducer.

The first transducers were single, flat crystals that radiated planar waves. Most current transducers are composed of several narrow piezoelectric elements arranged in a linear array. Annular arrays are ring-shaped and arranged concentrically. Contemporary phased-array transducers generally contain 64–128 narrow crystals, which produce a beam by firing the elements grouping a specific order. If a single element were fired, the beam pattern would be essentially circular in its radiation (Figure 1.7). By firing all the elements, it is possible to focus the beam, directing the ultrasound in any direction within a wide sector coplanar with the array (Figure 1.8). It is even possible to stimulate the array to send out multiple ultrasound pulses simultaneously in different directions, significantly improving ultrasound frame rates by processing multiple scan lines in parallel. Recently, transducer technology has been expanded to 2D arrays of crystals, allowing ultrasound pulses to be directed anywhere in a pyramid-shaped volume below the transducer, facilitating real-time 3D imaging.

When a reflected echo strikes the transducer, the piezoelectric crystal produces a miniscule voltage in response to the vibrations from the returning ultrasound. The returning echoes from shallow structures are as much as one billion-fold stronger than those from deeper layers, due to attenuation within

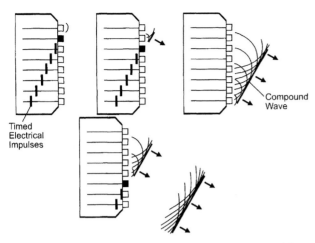

Figure 1.7 *Phased array echo transducer. It is possible to steer a planar ultrasound wave by changing the timing of transmission from a linear array of crystals. (Adapted from Topol EJ (ed.) Textbook of Cardiovascular Medicine, 2nd edn. Philadelphia: Lippincott, Williams and Wilkins, 2002:CD 46.5.1, with permission.)*

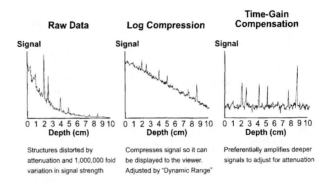

Figure 1.9 *Scan-line processing. Logarithmic compression and time-gain compensation is applied to the returning echoes to normalize the billion-fold variation in signal strength with depth. (Adapted from Topol EJ (ed.), Textbook of Cardiovascular Medicine, 2nd edn. Philadelphia: Lippincott, Williams and Wilkins, 2002:CD 46.5.3, with permission.)*

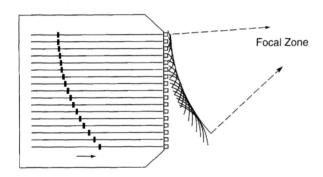

Figure 1.8 *Focused phased-array echo transducer. It is possible to focus the wavefront at a specific depth if the time delay between adjacent crystals is not constant. (Adapted from Topol EJ (ed.), Textbook of Cardiovascular Medicine, 2nd edn. Philadelphia: Lippincott, Williams and Wilkins, 2002:CD 46.5.2, with permission.)*

the tissues. Since the human eye can only appreciate about 100 Gy levels on the monitor, echo signals must be compressed to a smaller dynamic range by logarithmic amplification, which amplifies weak input signals much more than strong ones, in effect converting an exponential distribution of voltages into a linear one. Time-gain compensation is then applied to give greater amplification to echoes returning from deeper structures, adjusted by the user for individual variation in attenuation (Figure 1.9). The amplified signal now consists of the radiofrequency ultrasound wave, modulated in time by the reflections from the body. In most echo instruments, these lower-frequency

(100–500 kHz) modulations are extracted from the megahertz carrier by full-wave rectification and low-pass filtration, leaving only the amplitude of the ultrasonic reflections. Recently, however, it has become possible to use the phase information (in addition to the usual signal magnitude) to improve lateral resolution of the ultrasonic image, allowing objects to be localized even if they fall between the scan lines.

Ultrasound data can be displayed in a variety of scan formats. In M-mode echocardiography, repeated echo pulses are made along a single scan line, and the processed envelope is drawn vertically on the output video with subsequent envelopes displaced rightward, so that the horizontal axis of the display corresponds to time, whereas the vertical axis relates to distance from the transducer. The M-mode is used to make precise axial measurements and view rapidly moving structures, but is not often used in ICE due to the difficulty of maintaining orientation from the unidirectional image (Figure 1.10).

More useful for catheter guidance is the sector or 2D scan format, where a fan of scan lines originate from a common point, creating a shape much like a pie wedge. Echo interrogations are made sequentially throughout a 60–90° sector, with about 100 scan lines per frame. For example, at a 20 cm imaging depth, pulses can be emitted every 260 µs, allowing 100 scan lines per frame to be formed in 26 ms, and a display rate of over 38 frames per second. With parallel processing, up to four scan lines can be displayed simultaneously, allowing frame rates over 150 per second (Figure 1.11).

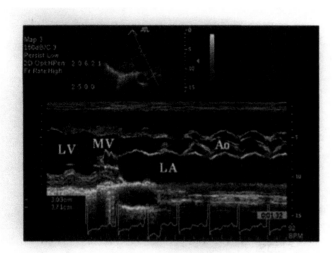

Figure 1.10 *M-mode echocardiographic imaging. The M-mode display shows time horizontally and depth vertically. Ao, aorta; LA, left atrium; LV, left ventricle; MV, mitral valve. (From Topol EJ (ed.), Textbook of Cardiovascular Medicine, 2nd edn. Philadelphia: Lippincott, Williams and Wilkins, 2002:CD 46.6, with permission.)*

• Sound transmitted from a moving object:

$$\frac{\Delta f}{f} = \frac{v}{c}$$

• Sound transmitted from a moving object:

$$\frac{\Delta f}{f} = \frac{2v}{c}$$

• ...from an object moving at angle Θ

$$\frac{\Delta f}{f} = \frac{2v \cos \Theta}{c}$$

• Rearranging...

$$v = \frac{c \, \Delta f}{2f \cos \Theta}$$

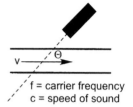

f = carrier frequency
c = speed of sound

Figure 1.12 *Principles of the Doppler shift. The frequency is shifted in proportion to the velocity when sound is emitted from a moving object. The factor 2 for reflected sound occurs because this shift occurs on absorption and reflection. Only the component of velocity parallel to the sound wave plays a factor in the Doppler shift. (Adapted from Topol EJ (ed.), Textbook of Cardiovascular Medicine, 2nd edn. Philadelphia: Lippincott, Williams and Wilkins, 2002:CD 46.9, with permission.)*

Serial Processing

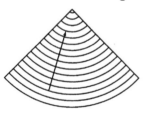

One scan line is received for each ultrasound pulse

Parallel Processing

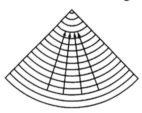

Several scan lines are received for each ultrasound pulse

Figure 1.11 *Serial versus parallel processing. Frame rate can be substantially improved by analyzing several scan lines simultaneously through parallel processing. (Adapted from Topol EJ (ed.), Textbook of Cardiovascular Medicine, 2nd edn. Philadelphia: Lippincott, Williams and Wilkins, 2002:CD 46.7, with permission.)*

The heart is actually a 4D structure, comprising three spatial dimensions of shape and one temporal dimension of motion. Spatial resolution reflects the smallest separation at which two objects can be distinguished and is not constant across the field of view with ultrasonography. Echocardiography has greater resolution in the near field than in the far field because of beam divergence, although this can be modified by focusing the beam. Furthermore, resolution in echocardiography is anisotropic: i.e. it is better in the axial direction (along the scan line) than in the lateral direction (across the scan line). One must also take care to distinguish the physical resolution of the imaging modality from the resolution of a video or computer screen. The spacing of the picture elements (pixels) on the screen may be greater or lesser than the physical resolution. This screen resolution typically is stated in the number of pixels across the screen in the horizontal and vertical direction. Overall spatial resolution is obviously the lesser of physical and screen resolutions. Temporal resolution reflects the frequency with which the image is generated, usually stated in frames per second. There is often a trade-off between temporal and spatial resolution. Echocardiograms can be generated more frequently; this usually requires that the density of scan lines per image be reduced, thus sacrificing image quality.

The ICE system is also able to quantify blood velocity via the Doppler principle, adding immensely to the value of echocardiography (Figure 1.12). Doppler imaging is based on the observation that sound reflected from a moving object is frequency-shifted in proportion to the ratio of the object velocity v and the sound velocity c:

$$f_{\mathrm{d}} = 2vf_{\mathrm{o}}/c$$

where f_{o} is the transducer frequency and f_{d} is the Doppler shift. The factor 2 occurs because the frequency is shifted when the sound hits the moving particle and again when it is re-radiated by scattering. Only particles that are parallel to the ultrasound beam affect the Doppler shift. For a particle moving at an angle θ to the scan line, the Doppler shift is proportional to the cosine of θ. Fo example, 30° misalignment leads to a 13% velocity underestimation.[5]

There are three basic ways the Doppler signal can be processed and displayed, each with its particular advantages and disadvantages. The first of these, pulsed-wave Doppler, measures a defined sample of blood flow by directing brief (1–4 μs) bursts of ultrasound into the patient. The receiver is timed to "listen" to the returning signal at a specific time delay and then processed by Fourier analysis to display velocity at a specific location. A limitation of pulsed-wave Doppler is its inability to display very high velocities, as a result of the phenomenon of aliasing, whereby the velocity display will suddenly wrap-around and appear to be going in the opposite velocity – much like how wagon wheels appear to be turning backward in the motion pictures (Figure 1.13). This arises because of the finite velocity of sound (c), which limits the rate at which pulses can be directed to a specific depth d, termed the pulse repetition velocity:

$$PRF = c/2d \quad \text{or} \quad 77/d$$

where d is in cm and PRF is expressed in kHz. Since a Doppler shift f_d must be interrogated twice per cycle, we can use the Doppler equation to relate this maximal (or Nyquist velocity v_N) to image depth and frequency:

$$v_N = c^2/8df_o$$

or approximately $35/df_o$, where v_N is in m/s, d is in cm, and f_o is in MHz. Thus, aliasing is a result of signals being undersampled and appearing misdirected. If one is certain of the direction of blood flow, one can shift the Doppler baseline and effectively double the velocity that can be displayed.

Continuous-wave (CW) Doppler differs from pulsed-wave Doppler in that the transducer is constantly emitting and receiving ultrasound. CW Doppler has no limitation on PRF and thus can accurately measure the elevated flow velocities seen in stenotic and regurgitant lesions. It cannot precisely determine the location of these velocities, but since they generally occur in only a few places within the heart, this isn't a major limitation (Figure 1.14).

Color flow Doppler superimposes color onto an echo sector scan to demonstrate the dynamic nature and distribution of velocity throughout the heart. Color Doppler is a valuable tool for assessing blood flow in both normal and pathologic conditions such as valvular regurgitation, stenosis, and various shunt lesions (Figure 1.15). It uses autocorrelation to measure the mean Doppler shift information and then simultaneously displays the 2D image with red representing flow towards the transducer and blue for flow away. Because color Doppler is derived from brief pulses of ultrasound, it suffers from

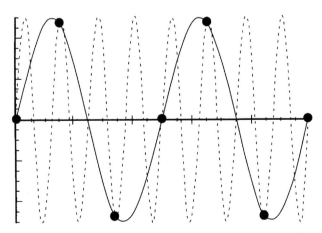

Figure 1.13 *Aliasing effect in Doppler echocardiography. If the actual Doppler waveform (dotted line) is undersampled* (white dots), *the reconstructed waveform (solid line) will be at a falsely low frequency (and thereby velocity). (Adapted from Topol EJ (ed.), Textbook of Cardiovascular Medicine, 2nd edn. Philadelphia: Lippincott, Williams and Wilkins, 2002:CD 46.9.3, with permission.)*

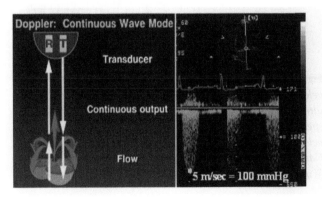

Figure 1.14 *Continuous wave Doppler. It is possible to quantify velocities of any magnitude by continuously transmitting and receiving Doppler-shifted echoes; however, this is at the cost of not having range information as to the specific depth of that velocity. A common application is quantification of aortic stenosis (right panel), using the simplified Bernoulli equation, $\Delta p = 4v^2$. (From Topol EJ (ed.), Textbook of Cardiovascular Medicine, 2nd edn. Philadelphia: Lippincott, Williams and Wilkins, 2002:CD 46.9.1, with permission.)*

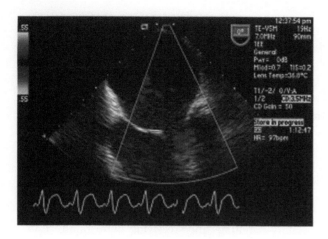

Figure 1.15 *Color Doppler echocardiography. It is possible to map velocity throughout the imaging sector by processing successive ultrasound pulses with autocorrelation techniques. (From Topol EJ (ed.), Textbook of Cardiovascular Medicine, 2nd edn. Philadelphia: Lippincott, Williams and Wilkins, 2002:CD 46.9.4, with permission.)*

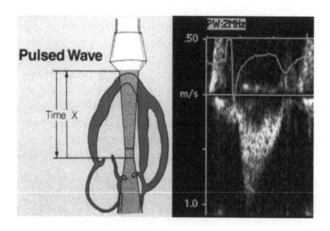

Figure 1.16 *Pulsed-wave Doppler. It is possible to localize velocities within the heart by transmitting a brief pulse of ultrasound and "listening" for returning echoes from a specific depth; however, being able to quantify very high velocities is limited. (From Topol EJ (ed.), Textbook of Cardiovascular Medicine, 2nd edn. Philadelphia: Lippincott, Williams and Wilkins, 2002:CD 46.18, with permission.)*

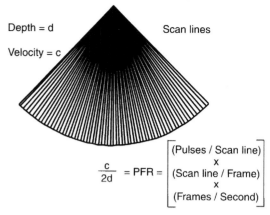

Figure 1.17 *Temporal, spatial, and velocity trade-offs in Doppler flow mapping. The pulse repetition frequency (PRF, number of interrogations per second) is fixed by the depth of imaging and the velocity of sound: PRF = c/2d. This PRF must be divided between the number of pulses per scan line (which determines velocity resolution), the number of scan lines per frame (which determines spatial extent and resolution of the flow map), and the number of frames per second (which is temporal resolution). (Adapted from Fozzard HA et al (eds), The Heart and Cardiovascular System, 2nd edn. New York: Raven, 1992:638, and from Topol EJ (ed.), Textbook of Cardiovascular Medicine, 2nd edn. Philadelphia: Lippincott, Williams and Wilkins, 2002:CD 46.21, with permission.)*

INDICATIONS, CONTRAINDICATIONS, AND THE RATIONALE FOR IMPLEMENTING INTRACARDIAC ECHOCARDIOGRAPHY IN INTERVENTIONAL ELECTROPHYSIOLOGY

Phased-array intracardiac echocardiography has proven to be a valuable tool in evaluating cardiac structures and for directing therapeutic interventions in a variety of rhythm disorders, valve dysfunction, and structural abnormalities.[1,2] The potential advantages of ICE-guided ablations have been assessed both for atrial and ventricular arrhythmias. Additionally, ICE guidance has been used to detect pacemaker lead vegetation in patients with endocarditis and to facilitate pacemaker laser lead extraction.[2] ICE has been able to overcome the visualization limitations associated with fluoroscopy and to precisely target areas such as the pulmonary veins, crista terminalis, the Eustachian ridge, the tricuspid annulus, and the coronary sinus ostium.[1,2,6] The influence of ICE has been most prominently noted during ablation of atrial

the same aliasing limits as pulsed-wave Doppler (Figure 1.16). Furthermore, since each scan line must be pulsed 4–8 times to estimate velocity accurately, the frame rate in color Doppler is considerably lower than that of 2D Doppler. As mentioned above, however, parallel processing of multiple scan lines simultaneously can improve frame rate significantly (Figure 1.17).

fibrillation. ICE allows direct imaging of key sites, thus allowing for shortened fluoroscopy times. It also facilitates transseptal puncture by providing excellent visualization of the interatrial septum as well as the Brockenbrough needle tenting and traversing the fossa ovalis membrane.[2,7] The ability to visualize these structures during transseptal puncture has helped avoid complications and alleviate fear associated with this procedure.[2] The implementation of ICE decreases the likelihood of complications that are associated with transseptal puncture, such as aortic root puncture and left atrial perforation.[1,2]

Successful isolation of the PVs is dependent upon having good contact between the ablation tip and the endocardial surface. Inadequate contact between the tissue and the catheter reduces the amount of heat transmitted to the endocardial surface and allows dissipation of heat into the circulating blood, resulting in poor lesion formation and an increased likelihood of clot formation. ICE is able to provide the operator with accurate visualization of the catheter–cardiac tissue interface, detection of catheter migration, and identification of thrombus formation.[1,2]

In most radiofrequency ablation procedures, temperature, power, and impedance are monitored. When tissue is superheated, a rise in impedance occurs. This superheating can lead to microbubbles at the ablation site and can lead to possible char formation or thrombus on the catheter and an increased risk of PV stenosis.[2] These microbubbles represent blood gases being driven out of solution, steam, and particles of disrupted tissue and coagulated blood.[1,5] When scattered microbubbles are located adjacent to the length of the catheter, immediate lowering or discontinuation of radiofrequency delivery reduces the likelihood that patients will have PV stenosis, pericardial effusion, cerebral embolism, or atria esophageal fistula. This protocol reduces the likelihood that patients will have PV stenosis, perforation, pericardial effusion, cerebral embolism, or atrio-esophageal fistula.[8,9] Consequently, ICE is able to optimize energy titration during radiofrequency energy delivery through the detection of bubbles at the catheter–tissue interface.

ICE can also be used to monitor complications immediately. Early detection of char or thrombus formation can alert the operator to remove the catheter, thereby reducing the likelihood of cerebral embolism.[2,8,9] Current ICE systems include real-time color Doppler, which allows the operator to monitor PV ostial narrowing during the procedure. It also allows for rapid evaluation and treatment of pericardial effusion/tamponade.

LIMITATIONS IN USING INTRACARDIAC ECHOCARDIOGRAPHY AS A CLINICAL TOOL

One drawback of the technique is that it remains an invasive means of visualizing the heart. Furthermore, ICE cannot provide multiple planar visualization in a wide view.[1,2,7] Another constraint is the relatively large size of the catheter (10F) required to house a linear phased-array transducer, thus limiting it to venous applications.[1] However, smaller 8F catheters have recently been released. Finally, the cost of using the ICE catheters remains high, which makes it difficult financially for all institutions to implement.[1,2]

Nevertheless, there is a strong rationale for incorporating ICE into interventional electrophysiologic procedures, because it provides better visualization, fewer complications, better success rates (due to accurate assessment of location and good catheter–endocardium contact), and shortened fluoroscopy times. ICE allows a single operator to manage both the imaging and therapeutic catheter, while providing the ability to assess real-time hemodynamics via color Doppler.[1,2] However, perhaps the best rationale for the implementation of ICE in interventional electrophysiology is that it is a great equalizer. It has simplified procedures and reduced complications, even in relatively inexperienced hands, and thus has allowed more electrophysiologists to perform procedures previously limited to tertiary care institutions.

REFERENCES

1. Packer DL, Stevens CL, Curley MG, et al. Intracardiac phased-array imaging: methods and initial clinical experience with high resolution, under blood visualization: initial experience with phased-array ultrasound. J Am Cardiol 2002; 39: 509–16.

2. Hynes BJ, Mart C, Atman S, et al. Role of intracardiac ultrasound in interventional electrophysiology. Curr Opin Cardiol 2004; 19: 52–7.

3. Foster G, Picard M. Intracardiac echocardiography: current uses and future directions. Echocardiography 2001; 18: 43–8.

4. Smith SW, Light ED, Idriss SF, Wolf PD. Feasibility study of real-time three-dimensional intracardiac echocardiography for guidance of interventional electrophysiology. Pacing Clin Electrophysiol 2002; 25: 351–7.

5. Wood MA, Shaffer KM, Ellenbogen AL, Ownby ED. Microbubbles during radiofrequency catheter ablation: composition and formation. Heart Rhythm 2005; 2(4): 397–403.

6. Carlo L, Lamberti F, et al. Intracardiac echocardiography: from electroanatomic correlation to clinical application in interventional electrophysiology. Ital Heart J 2002; 3: 387–98.

7. Bruce CJ, Friedman PA. Intracardiac echocardiography. Echocardiography 2001; 2: 234–44.

8. Marrouche N, Martin D, Wazni O, et al. Phased-array intracardiac echocardiography monitoring during pulmonary vein isolation in patients with atrial fibrillation: impact on outcome and complications. Circulation 2003; 107: 2710–16.

9. Pappone C, Oral H, Santinelli V, et al. Atrio-esophageal fistula as a complication of percutaneous transcatheter ablation of atrial fibrillation. Circulation 2004; 109: 2724–6.

Chapter 2   **Atrial chambers: gross anatomy and intracardiac phased-array echocardiography imaging**

Sakis Themistoclakis, Aldo Bonso, Antonio Rossillo, and Antonio Raviele

INTRODUCTION

Intracardiac echocardiography (ICE) images the heart with only slight movements of the catheter. Recent advances in image reconstruction with phased-array ultrasound catheters have allowed for an enhanced assessment of cardiac anatomy, thereby improving the quality of information obtained and reducing the difficulty associated with certain procedures. Nevertheless, the ability to accurately assess and image cardiac structures is dependent upon one's understanding of the cardiac anatomy. Therefore, the first section of this chapter will focus on some basic anatomic landmarks which are useful to navigate ablation catheters.

ANATOMY

GROSS HEART

The long axis of the heart is obliquely positioned within the body. In the coronal plane, the right cardiac chambers are more anterior in relation to their left counterparts.[1] The atrial chambers are located slightly posterior and to the right of their respective ventricle.[1] Both right and left atria have an appendage, a venous component, and a vestibule. The two chambers are separated by the interatrial septum.

THE RIGHT ATRIUM

The large right atrial appendage is triangular with a broad base.[2-4] The right appendage dominates the right atrium. Its walls are lined with pectinate muscles which extend like the teeth of a comb from the terminal crest to reach anterior to the smooth-walled vestibule that surrounds the tricuspid valve orifice. Extending anteriorly and superiorly, the tip of the right appendage points left to overlie the root of the aorta.[2-4] The rest of the pectinated appendage forms the entire anterior right atrial wall; therefore, it is a mistake to consider only the tip as a representation of the right appendage.[2] The junction between the right appendage and smooth-walled venous component is marked internally by the prominent crista terminalis, which corresponds externally with the terminal groove. The terminal crest extends laterally and inferiorly under the orifice of the superior vena cava as a C-shaped structure ramifying as the pectinate muscles fan out anteriorly to insert at the vestibule of the tricuspid valve.[2-4]

The systemic venous components include the inferior vena cava (IVC), superior vena cava (SVC) and the coronary sinus (CS). The SVC and the IVC enter the right atrium in an obtuse angle. The SVC is situated anterior to the IVC. The right upper pulmonary vein passes behind the superior cavoatrial junction, whereas the lower pulmonary vein passes behind the intercaval area.[2] The sinus node is located between the junction of the superior vena cava and the terminal groove. The remnants of the right venous valve, the Eustachian valve, and the Thebesian valve are attached to the terminal crest, with the pectinate muscles (Eustachian ridge) extending in parallel fashion from the crest to run all around the vestibule, separating the smooth-walled venous sinus from the vestibule.[3] The inferior cavotricuspid isthmus is defined as the part of the lower right atrium located lateral and inferior to the coronary sinus ostium, and is limited posteriorly by the Eustachian valve/Eustachian ridge and anteriorly by the hinge of the septal leaflet.[2-5] The lateral boundary of the cavotricuspid isthmus is formed by the trabeculated free wall of the right atrium. This zone of slow conduction, represented by a pattern of abundant crossover and interlacing muscle bundles, is crucial for the genesis of typical atrial flutter. The posterior portion of the isthmus tends to be thin-walled and fibrotic, whereas the mid portion is trabeculated and the anterior portion smooth.[2] The posterior two portions of the isthmus often form a pouch, the sub-Eustachian pouch, which is located anterior to the Eustachian valve. The Eustachian valve[2] has great anatomic variations, ranging from being large to virtually absent and from being muscular to membrane-like. Similarly, the Thebesian valve, which guards the orifice of the coronary sinus, varies morphologically among individuals.[2] The Eustachian ridge, containing the tendon of Todaro, is a fibrous structure that continues directly with the free margin of the Eustachian valve. It separates the orifice of the inferior vena cava from the coronary sinus. The tendon of Todaro courses under the Eustachian ridge toward the central fibrous body. It ends at the junction between the atrioventricular node and the His bundle or directly above the His bundle.[2-5] The Eustachian ridge and the attachment of the septal leaflet of the tricuspid valve mark the lateral margins of the triangle of Koch. The triangle of Koch is defined as the inferior paraseptal right atrial region containing the atrioventricular node. The base of the triangle is composed of the orifice of the coronary sinus and the vestibular region, which extends from the coronary sinus to the tricuspid valve. The His bundle is generally located at the vertex of the Koch triangle.[3]

INTERATRIAL SEPTUM

In a sense, the true interatrial septum can be excised without exiting the heart. The interatrial septum is composed of the flap valve and the oval fossa. The fossa ovalis is an oval depression in the inferior right atrial septum which is traditionally considered to be the interatrial septum. The rest of the muscular interatrial septum is a deep infolding of the atrial walls with the exception of antero-inferior rim that anchors the flap valve to the antrioventricular junction.[2-6] This area, which is better described as the interatrial groove, is filled with fibrofatty tissue which is continuous with the extracardiac fat and frequently contains the artery supplying the sinus node. When a transseptal catheterization is required, it is important to perform the puncture at the level of the oval fossa. A puncture through the interatrial groove may result in a hemopericardium, especially in patients who are highly anticoagulated. The blood will dissect the fibrofatty tissue that is sandwiched in this virtual cavity between the right and left atrial myocardium.[3]

In about 25% of adult hearts the valve of the oval fossa remains separate from the anterosuperior rim of the fossa. This crevice allows for direct access to the left atrium without transseptal puncture.[3,6]

LEFT ATRIUM

The internal body of the left atrium (LA) is smooth. The only trabeculated portion is the left atrial appendage. The four pulmonary veins (PVs) drain into the left atrium.[2-6] Excluding the atrial appendage, the left atrium is composed of 4 walls which are described as superior, anterior, posterior, and left lateral. The anterior wall, located behind the transverse pericardial sinus, is very thin. Ho et al observed that the median thickness of the anterior, posterior, superior, and lateral left atrial walls were 3, 4, 4.5, and 4 mm, respectively.[6]

The vestibule is the smooth circumferential area that surrounds the orifice of the mitral valve. This is the thinnest left atrial area, with a median transmural thickness of 2 mm.[6] The posterior portion of the vestibular component is situated directly opposite the wall of the coronary sinus. Just proximal to the vestibular component, the left atrial wall is usually smooth. Unlike the right atrium, the left atrium is without an array of pectinate muscles. On the left side, the pectinate muscles are contained mostly within the atrial appendage.[2-6]

The left appendage is a true diverticulum. It is located superiorly and anteriorly to the orifice of the left superior pulmonary vein, pointing toward the aortic root. A narrow mouth marks the junction between the appendage and the venous component. At times, it produces a pronounced shelf between the appendage and left pulmonary veins.[2-6]

The venous component, consisting of the four pulmonary veins, represents a major part of the left atrium. The four pulmonary veins, which drain the blood from the left and right lung, are called the left superior, the left inferior, the right superior, and the right inferior pulmonary veins. However, anatomic variants are common and can be detected with computed tomography (CT) scan or magnetic resonance imaging (MRI) in more than 50% of cases. Common anatomic variants include a common ostium of the PVs and supernumerary veins.[7,8] The common veins are defined as the coalescence of superior and inferior veins proximal to the junction of the left atrial body.[8] Supernumerary veins are additional (neither superior nor inferior) vein(s) having an independent atriovenous junction. Another variant is represented by an ostial branch of the pulmonary vein defined as a PV branch joining within 5 mm of the atriovenous junction.[8] The supernumerary veins are commonly located on the right. They mainly drain the middle lobe of the lung and less frequently the superior segment of the lobe of the lung. Conversely, they are rarely detected on the left (25% vs 3%).[8] A common pulmonary vein is detected frequently on the left (up to 30%)[7] and can be characterized by a short or long common trunk (22% vs 7%).[7] The incidence of PV ostial branching is up to 66%, and is significantly higher on the right than on the left PV. They are more commonly seen in inferior rather than superior pulmonary veins.[8]

In general, the PV ostia are neither circular nor planar. The PVs are oblong, with the anteroposterior diameter of the PV ostia being less than the superoinferior dimension.[8,9] The ostia of the inferior PVs are more posterior and medial compared with those of the superior PVs. The "antrum" of the left and right PVs is defined as the funnel-shaped area proximal to the tube-like portion of the PVs. The orifices of the left PVs are located more superiorly than those on the right. The right superior PVs and the left superior PVs project forward and upward, whereas the right inferior PVs and the left inferior PVs project backward and downward. The right superior PVs lie just behind the superior vena cava and are situated adjacent to the plane of the atrial septum. The left PVs are positioned between the left appendage and the descending aorta. The ostium of the left superior PV lies in close proximity to the left appendage and is located just superior and posterior to its orifice.[8] The left PVs have a longer "neck", with a greater distance between the ostium and the first branch than the right PVs.[7]

IMAGING MODALITIES

Currently, a variety of imaging modalities are used to visualize the atrial chambers. These include MRI, CT, transesophageal echocardiography (TEE), angiography or fluoroscopy, and intracardiac echocardiography (ICE). Wood et al compared the defined PV ostial anatomy using all these imaging techniques in 24 patients with atrial fibrillation having radiofrequency catheter ablation. They observed that CT accurately identified the greatest number of PV ostia, followed by ICE. Moreover, angiography overestimates and TEE underestimates ostial diameters in

comparison with CT or ICE.[10] During the electrophysiologic (EP) procedure, cardiac chambers can be visualized in real time, only with angiography, fluoroscopy, or ICE; ICE is more accurate than the other two in the identification of important anatomic structures such as the crista terminalis, cardiac valve, oval fossa, and venous structures. In particular, Marrouche et al compared the PV ostium, defined angiographically and under ICE guidance on 125 PVs. The PV ostium, defined angiographically, was found to correlate with the ICE-defined PV ostium in only 15% of PVs, whereas in 85% of PVs ICE showed that the placement of the circular mapping catheter based on angiography was inaccurate and distal to the true LA–PV junction (5 ± 3 mm within the PV).[11] Furthermore, Schwartzman et al observed that there was complete concordance between multidimensional CT and phased-array ICE in discerning common and supernumerary veins as well as the ostial branches.[8]

INTRACARDIAC ECHOCARDIOGRAPHY IMAGING OF ATRIAL CHAMBERS

Acuson AcuNav[TM] Diagnostic Ultrasound catheter utilizes a phased array transducer, available in 8 or 10 French design mounted on a steerable deflectable catheter and can be used on a variety of Acuson~Siemens ultrasound systems including the Sequoia[TM], Aspen[TM] (10 French only), the Cypress[TM] and most recently the CV70[TM] (8 French only). The ICE catheter is inserted in the patient through a femoral vein approach, through an 11F hemostatic sheath, and is advanced via the inferior vena cava (IVC) and positioned in the right atrium (RA) or right ventricle (RV).[11–14] All the different views of the right and left atrium are obtained from the right chamber with gentle movements of the catheter. The initial view that the operator is looking for is called the "RA home view", which is used for orientation. This view, obtained with the ICE catheter positioned in the mid right atrium with the imaging head in an anterior direction without tip deflection, visualizes the right atrium, the tricuspid valve, and the right ventricle long axis (Figure 2.1). From the RA home view, slight counterclockwise rotation by 10–15° allows for visualization of the crista terminalis with pectinate muscles (Figures 2.2, 2.3).[14] The right appendage comes into view with continued counterclockwise rotation. Posterior deflection of the catheter may be required to optimize the visualization of the tip of the appendage (Figure 2.4).

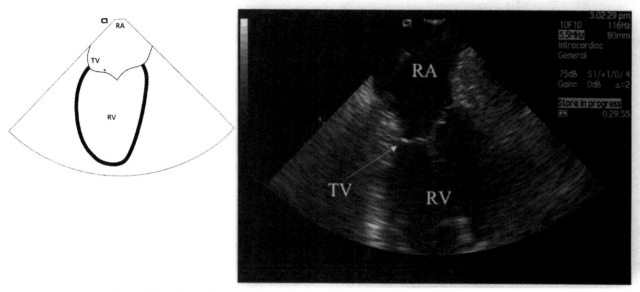

Figure 2.1 *Home View. RA, right atrium; TV, tricuspid valve; RV, right ventricle.*

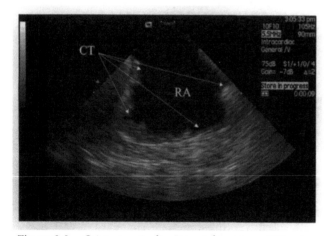

Figure 2.2 *Crista terminalis. RA, right atrium; CT, crista terminalis.*

Clockwise catheter rotation from the terminal crista to the RA home view, at the level of the RA–IVC junction or immediately above, visualizes the cavotricuspid isthmus, with its anterior and posterior boundaries comprising tricuspid valve and Eustachian ridge with the remnant Eustachian valve, respectively (Figure 2.5).[15] Clockwise rotation brings the coronary sinus ostium into view as medial or septal boundary of the cavotricuspid isthmus (Figures 2.6a and 2.6b). Counterclockwise rotation allows visualization of the

latter boundary represented by the free wall of the left atrium.[15] Advancing the catheter from the home view in the high right atrium, with a posterior tilt of 30°, allows for visualization of the RA–SVC (superior vena cava) junction. The junction between the right atrium and the superior vena cava is marked by the border between the pulmonary artery and the interatrial septum (Figure 2.7). The clockwise rotation of the catheter of about 15–30° from the home view visualizes the RV outflow tract and aortic root (Figure 2.8). With further clockwise catheter rotation, the left atrium comes into view with interatrial septum and left atrial appendage (Figure 2.9). Backward deflection of the catheter tip moves the image further from the imaging head, whereas forward deflection of the tip moves the target closer. Therefore, sometimes a posterior tilt of the imaging tip may be required to optimize the visualization of the entire septum and the oval fossa (Figures 2.10a and 2.10b). The thin and flap membrane of the oval foramen can be clearly visualized; therefore, this view is very useful for the transseptal puncture. Indeed, the transseptal needle can be correctly positioned on the fossa ovalis and the transseptal puncture monitored. ICE allows visualization of the needle initially tenting the oval fossa and then crossing through the septum in the LA (Figure 2.10c). With a slight clockwise rotation of the catheter, it is possible to scan the entire interatrial septum from anterior to posterior. Visualization of the transseptal sheath in the

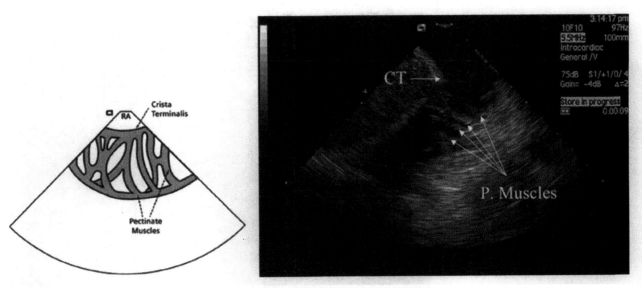

Figure 2.3 *Crista terminalis with pectinate muscles. RA, right atrium; CT, crista terminalis; P. Muscles, pectinate muscles.*

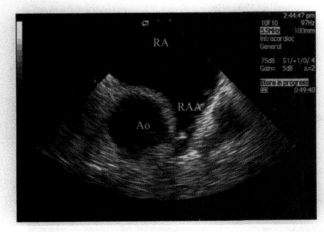

Figure 2.4 *Right atrial appendage. RA, right atrium; Ao, aorta; RAA, right atrial appendage.*

same view as the left pulmonary veins, safely directs the transseptal sheath towards the posterior wall of the left atrium (Figure 2.10d). The transseptal puncture at this site facilitates navigation of the catheters around the pulmonary veins. From the interatrial septum view, slight advancement of the catheter, or minimal tilting of the catheter tip posteriorly, and adjusting the depth control to around 100 mm, allows visualization of the left superior and left inferior pulmonary veins in the long-axis view (Figure 2.11a). Color Doppler can be utilized to identify these veins. The movement of blood from these veins is towards the transducer, therefore,

the color Doppler flow is red (Figures 2.11b-1, 2.11b-2, and 2.11b-3). It is not unusual to observe a common ostium of the left pulmonary veins with a long or short common trunk (Figures 2.12, 2.13a, 2.13b, and 2.13c). A counterclockwise catheter rotation from this view visualizes the mitral valve and left appendage immediately anteriorly to the left superior PV (see Figure 2.9). Color Doppler can also be utilized to differentiate the appendage from the PVs. Clockwise rotation of the catheter past the left pulmonary veins, maintaining a neutral position, allows for visualization of the right pulmonary veins. The right superior and inferior pulmonary veins will appear in a cross-sectional view (Figure 2.14). To obtain the long-axis view, the catheter has to be deflected posteriorly. Usually, the long-axis view of right inferior PV appears first (Figures 2.15a and 2.15b). From this view, clockwise rotation of the catheter visualizes the long-axis view of the right superior PV (Figure 2.16a). The long-axis view of the right superior PV can be differentiated from the long-axis view of the right inferior PV by the presence of the long-axis view of the right branch of the pulmonary artery (Figures 2.16b-1 and 2.16b-2). The long-axis view of the right PVs allows for visualization of early branches or supranumerary veins (Figures 2.17a, 2.17b, 2.17c, 2.18a, 2.18b, and 2.18c). Color Doppler can be useful in these cases to identify the accessory veins (Figures 2.17a, 2.17b, 2.17c, 2.18a, 2.18b, and 2.18c). From the right superior long-axis view, tilting the catheter more posteriorly toward the ventricle in conjunction with a slight counterclockwise rotation

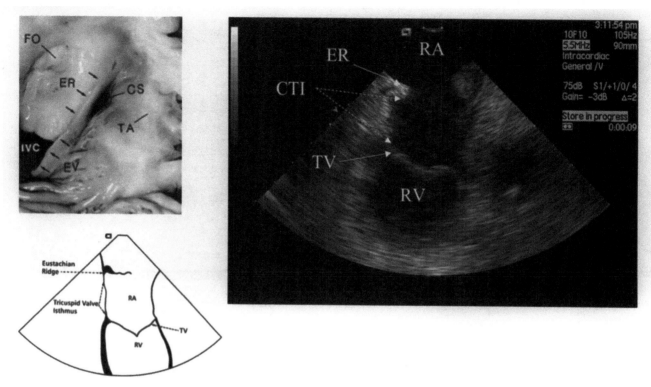

Figure 2.5 *Eustachian ridge and cavotricuspid isthmus. RA, right atrium; ER, Eustachian ridge; CTI, Cavotricuspid isthmus; TV, tricuspid valve; RV, right ventricle.*

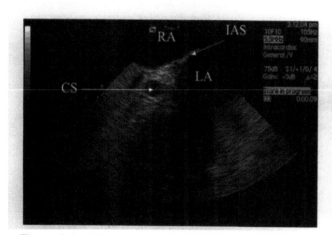

Figure 2.6a *Coronary sinus short-axis view. RA, right atrium; CS, coronary sinus; IAS, Interatrial septum; LA, left atrium.*

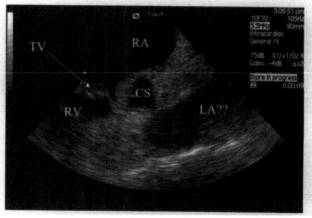

Figure 2.6b *Coronary sinus short-axis view. RA, right atrium; TV, tricuspid valve; CS, coronary sinus; RV, right ventricle; LA, left atrium.*

allows for visualization of the right and left superior PV along with the posterior wall of the LA (Figures 2.19a and 2.19b). In this view, the posterior extension of the antra of the pulmonary veins is shown. It is evident that on the posterior wall the right and left PV antra connect with each other. By tilting the catheter more posteriorly and advancing it in the right ventricle in conjunction with counterclockwise rotation, it is possible to visualize the left atrial appendage (Figures 2.20a and 2.20b). With further slight advancement of the catheter in the right ventricle, the right PV disappears, and the image of the left superior PV with the left appendage can be better seen (Figure 2.21). In this view the anterior segments of the left superior PV antrum are clearly defined as well as the pronounced shelf between the left superior PV and the appendage.

Finally, it is possible to measure by pulsed-wave or continuous-wave Doppler the flow in each pulmonary vein or in the appendage (Figures 2.22a, 2.22b, 2.22c, 2.22d, 2.22e, and 2.22f). Saad et al measured pulmonary vein blood flow with ICE immediately before and after the pulmonary vein isolation with radiofrequency ablation. They observed that the average preablation diastolic flows for the left superior, left inferior, right superior, and right inferior pulmonary veins were 0.56, 0.54, 0.47, and 0.45 m/s, respectively. These values increased significantly after the ablation procedure (0.74, 0.67, 0.58, and 0.59 m/s, respectively). However, these acute changes in the pulmonary vein flow, immediately after the ablation, did not predict subsequent development of chronic stenosis, as assessed by CT 3 months after the procedure.[15]

SUMMARY OF KEY POINTS

- Upon insertion of the catheter into the right atrium, with the notched handle markers upright, a small degree of counterclockwise rotation will result in imaging the Crista terminalis and the right atrial appendage.
- Rotating clockwise, back to the insertion position and slightly further clockwise, about 15–30°, will bring into view the tricuspid valve and the right ventricle. This is called the "Home View". There is no deflection on the catheter tip to visualize this.
- Continuing clockwise, about 30–40° from the 'Home View', will display the RVOT and pulmonic valve.
- Further clockwise rotation will bring the left ventricle into view and may include the aortic valve in the field of view.
- Further clockwise rotation, to a total of about 60–80° from 'Home' will bring into view the left ventricle, the mitral valve, the interatrial septum and the left atrial appendage.
- From here, further clockwise rotation will bring into view the left pulmonary veins, and if the catheter is slightly advance (inserted further into the heart) the fossa ovalis may be visualized. In many cases posterior and rightward flexion of the catheter tip will facilitate better visualization of the fossa for transseptal catheterization.
- With the catheter tip back in the neutral position, (deflection removed) further clockwise rotation will bring into view the right pulmonary veins in cross section. Further insertion plus a slight additional clockwise rotation and then posterior tilt will allow longitudinal visualization of the right superior vein.

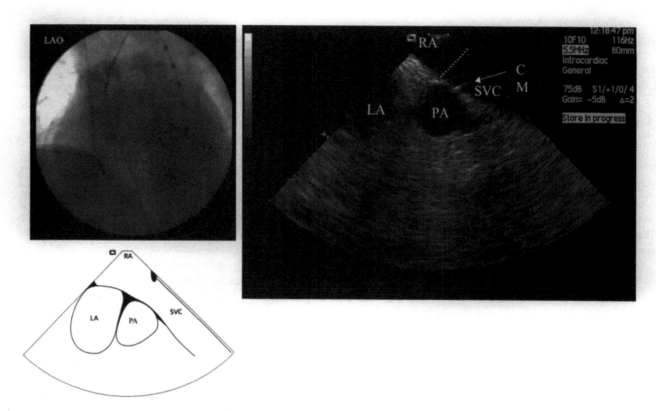

Figure 2.7   *Right atrium–superior vena cava junction. RA, right atrium; LA, left atrium; PA, pulmonary artery; SVC, superior vena cava; CM, circular mapping catheter. The RA–SVC junction is marked by the dotted yellow line.*

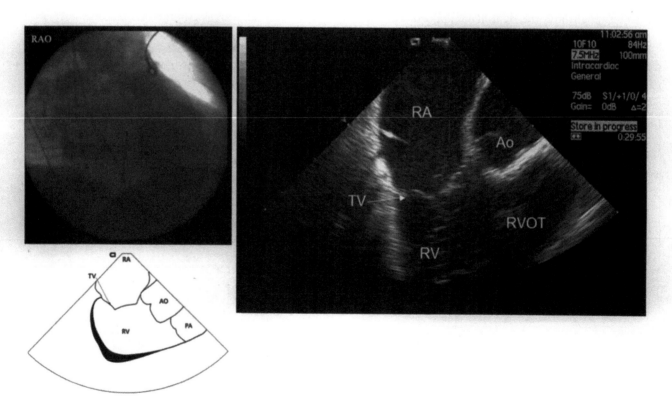

Figure 2.8   *Aorta and right ventricle outflow tract. RA, right atrium; TV, tricuspid valve; RV, right ventricle; RVOT, right ventricular outflow tract; Ao, aorta (long-axis view).*

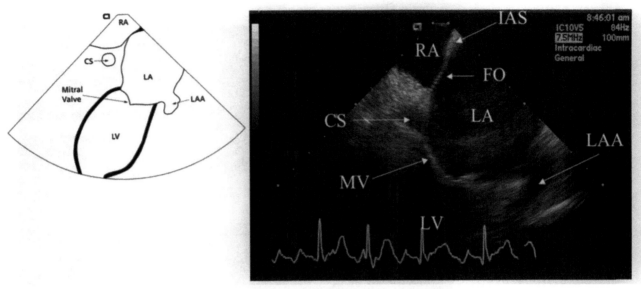

Figure 2.9 *Left atrial appendage. RA, right atrium; IAS, interatrial septum; FO, fossa ovalis; CS, coronary sinus; LA, left atrium; LV, left ventricle; LAA, left atrial appendage; MV, mitral value.*

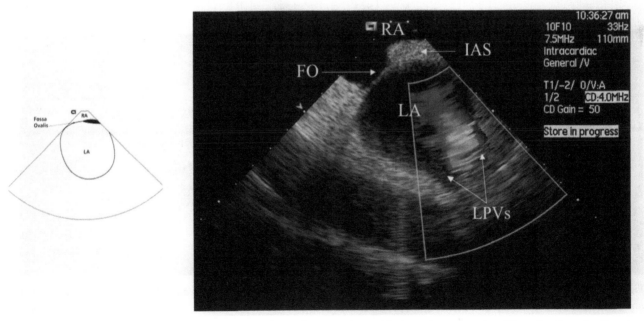

Figure 2.10a *Interatrial septum with the fossa ovalis in the same view with the pulmonary veins. The color Doppler flow is coming from the left superior pulmonary vein. RA, right atrium; FO, fossa ovalis; IAS, interatrial septum; LA, left atrium; LPVs, left pulmonary veins.*

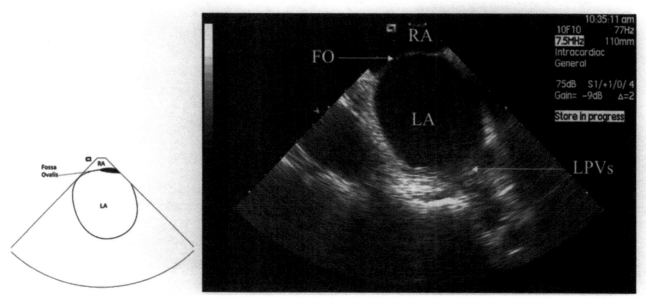

Figure 2.10b *Interatrial septum with fossa ovalis. RA, right atrium; FO, fossa ovalis; LA, left atrium; LPVs, left pulmonary veins.*

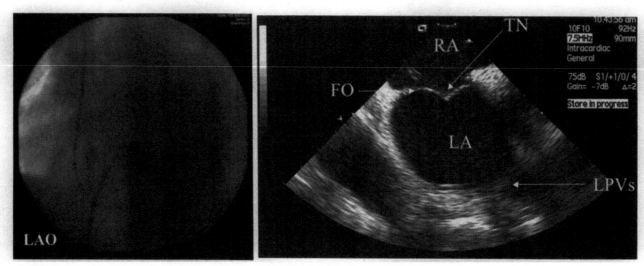

Figure 2.10c *Interatrial septum with fossa ovalis during transseptal puncture. RA, right atrium; FO, fossa ovalis; LA, left atrium; LPVs, left pulmonary veins; TN, transseptal needle.*

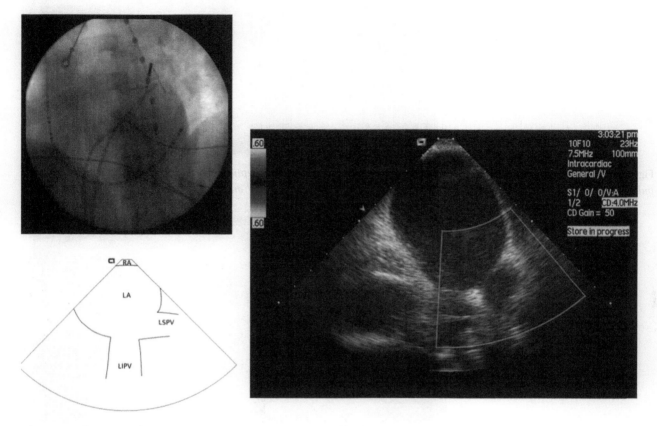

Figure 2.10d *RA, right atrium; LA, left atrium; LIPV, left inferior pulmonary vein; LSPV, left superior pulmonary vein.*

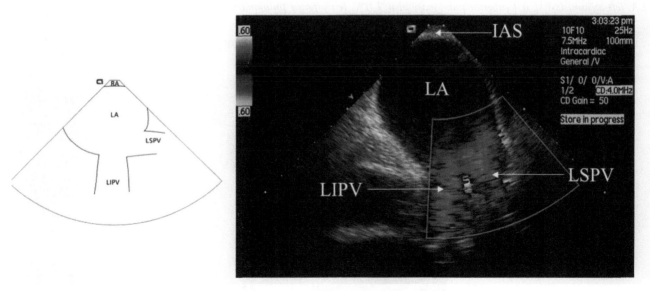

Figure 2.11a *Long-axis view of left pulmonary veins with color Doppler flow. IAS, Interatrial septum; LA, left atrium; LSPV, left superior pulmonary vein; LIPV, left inferior pulmonary vein; C, carina between the LSPV and LIPV.*

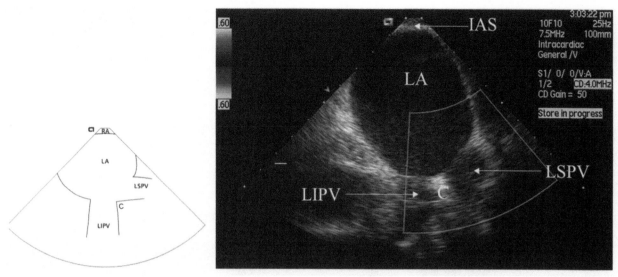

Figure 2.11b-1 *Long-axis view of the left pulmonary veins. IAS, interatrial septum; LA, left atrium; LSPV, left superior pulmonary vein; LIPV, left inferior pulmonary vein; C, carina between the LSPV and LIPV.*

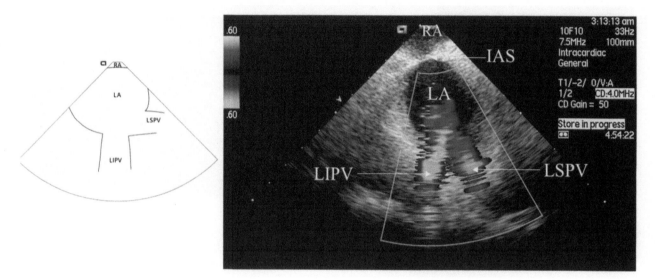

Figure 2.11b-2 *Long-axis view of the left pulmonary veins with Doppler color flow. RA, right atrium; IAS, interatrial septum; LA, left atrium; LSPV, left superior pulmonary vein; LIPV, left inferior pulmonary vein.*

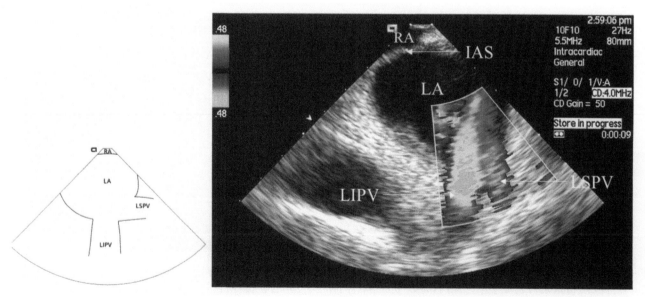

Figure 2.11b-3 *Long-axis view of the left pulmonary veins with color Doppler flow. RA, right atrium; IAS, interatrial septum; LA, left atrium; LSPV, left superior pulmonary vein; LIPV, left inferior pulmonary vein.*

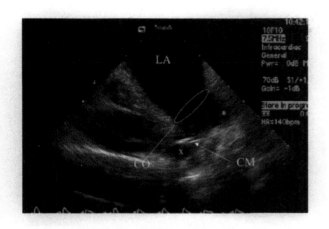

Figure 2.12 *Left pulmonary veins with common ostium and common trunk. LA, left atrium; CO, common ostium; CM, circular mapping catheter in the left inferior pulmonary vein; *, left superior pulmonary vein; x, left inferior pulmonary vein.*

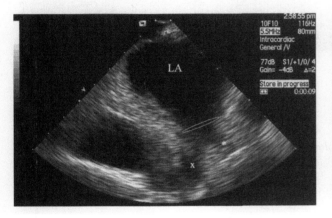

Figure 2.13a *Left pulmonary veins with short common ostium. LA, left atrium; circle, common ostium; *, left superior pulmonary vein; x, left inferior pulmonary vein.*

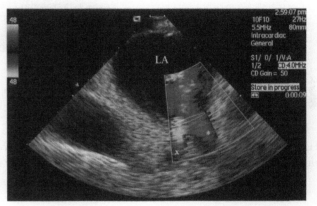

Figure 2.13b *Color Doppler flow from the left pulmonary veins with short common ostium. LA, left atrium; circle, short common ostium; *, left superior pulmonary vein; x, left inferior pulmonary vein.*

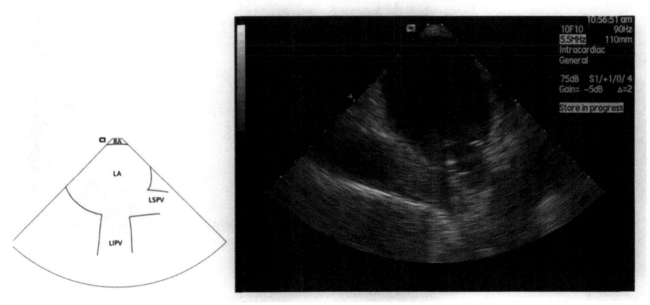

Figure 2.13c *Left superior and inferior pulmonary veins. RA, right atrium; LA, left ventricle; LSPV, left superior pulmonary vein; LIPV, left inferior pulmonary vein.*

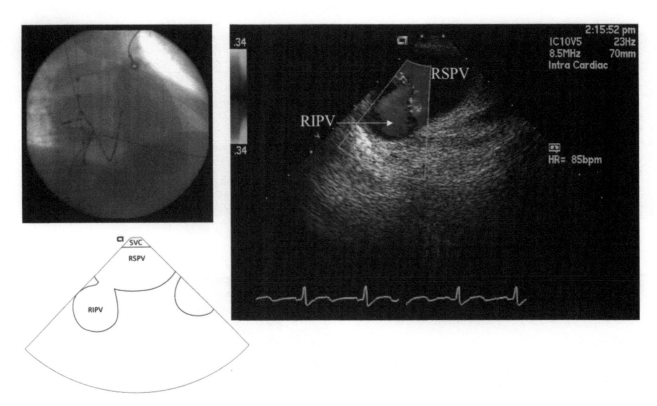

Figure 2.14   *Cross-sectional of the right pulmonary veins with color Doppler flow on the right inferior pulmonary vein. RSPV, right superior pulmonary vein; RIPV, right inferior pulmonary vein; SVC, superior vena cava.*

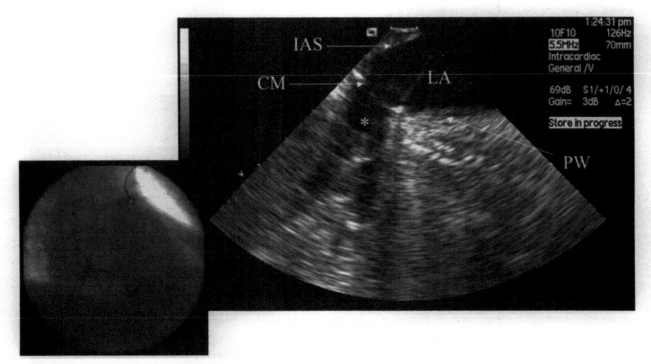

Figure 2.15a   *Long-axis view of the right inferior pulmonary vein with circular mapping catheter at left atrium–pulmonary vein junction. IAS, interatrial septum; *, right inferior pulmonary vein with two branches; LA, left atrium; CM, circular mapping catheter; PW, posterior wall of the left atrium.*

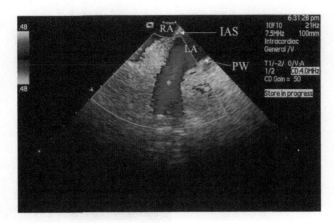

Figure 2.15b *Long-axis view of the right inferior pulmonary vein with Doppler flow. RA, right atrium; IAS, interatrial septum; *, right inferior pulmonary vein; LA, left atrium; PW, posterior wall of the left atrium.*

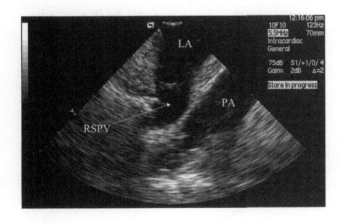

Figure 2.16a *Long-axis view of the right superior pulmonary vein. RSPV, right superior pulmonary vein; LA, left atrium; PA, right branch of pulmonary artery.*

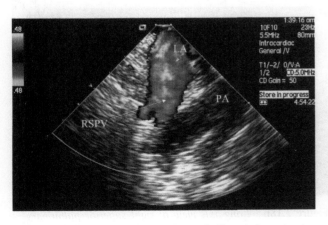

Figure 2.16b-1 *Long-axis view of the right superior pulmonary vein with color Doppler flow. RSPV, right superior pulmonary vein; LA, left atrium; PA, right branch of pulmonary artery.*

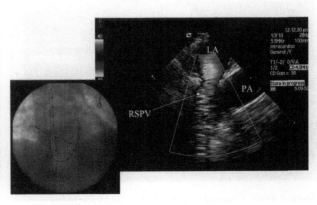

Figure 2.16b-2 *Long-axis view of right superior pulmonary vein with color Doppler flow. RSPV, right superior pulmonary vein; LA, left atrium; PA, right branch of pulmonary artery.*

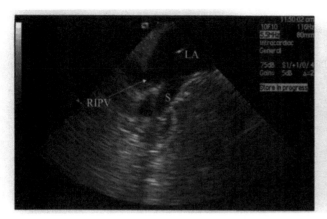

Figure 2.17a *Long-axis view of the right inferior pulmonary vein with early branching. RIPV, right inferior pulmonary vein with early branching; LA, left atrium; PW, posterior wall of the left atrium; S, supernumerary vein.*

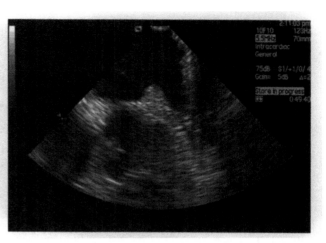

Figure 2.17c *Long-axis view of the right inferior pulmonary vein with supernumerary vein. RIPV, right inferior pulmonary vein; S, supranumerary vein; LA, left atrium.*

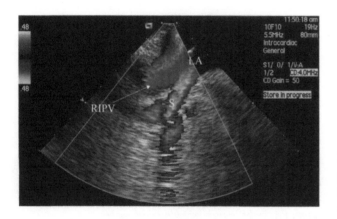

Figure 2.17b *Long-axis view of the right inferior pulmonary vein with supernumerary vein. RIPV, right inferior pulmonary vein; S, supranumerary vein; LA, left atrium.*

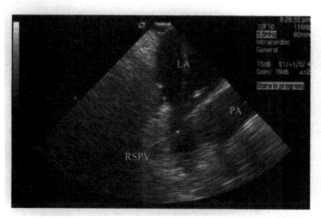

Figure 2.18a *Long-axis view of right superior pulmonary vein with early branching. RSPV, right superior pulmonary vein with early branching (*); LA, left atrium; PA, right branch of pulmonary artery.*

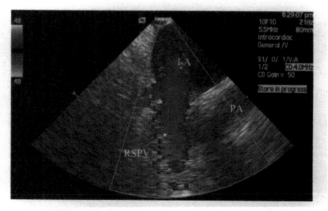

Figure 2.18b *Long-axis view of right superior pulmonary vein with early branching. RSPV, right superior pulmonary vein with early branching (*), LA, left atrium; PA, right branch of pulmonary artery.*

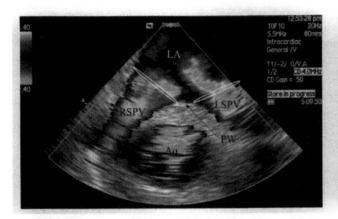

Figure 2.19a *Long-axis view of right and left superior pulmonary vein with PV antrum (color Doppler flow). RSPV, right superior pulmonary vein; LSPV, left superior pulmonary vein; LA, left atrium; Ao, descending aorta; PW, posterior left atrial wall; ellipse, antrum of pulmonary veins.*

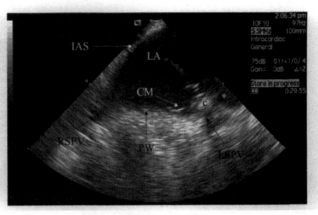

Figure 2.20a *Right superior pulmonary vein, left superior pulmonary vein, and left atrial appendage. RSPV, right superior pulmonary vein; CM, circular mapping catheter; *, left atrial appendage; c, carina between the left superior pulmonary vein and the appendage; LA, left atrium; IAS, interatrial septum; PW, posterior left atrial wall.*

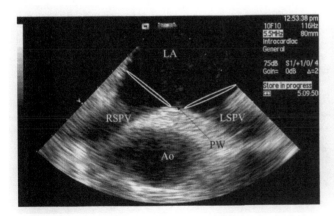

Figure 2.19b *Long-axis view of right and left superior pulmonary vein with PV antrum (color Doppler flow). RSPV, right superior pulmonary vein; LSPV, left superior pulmonary vein; LA, left atrium; Ao, descending aorta; PW, posterior left atrial wall; ellipse, antrum of pulmonary veins.*

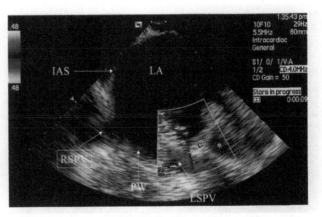

Figure 2.20b *Right superior pulmonary vein, left superior pulmonary vein, and left atrial appendage. RSPV, right superior pulmonary vein; CM, circular mapping catheter; *, left atrial appendage; c, carina between the left superior pulmonary vein and the appendage; LA, left atrium; IAS, interatrial septum; PW, posterior left atrial wall.*

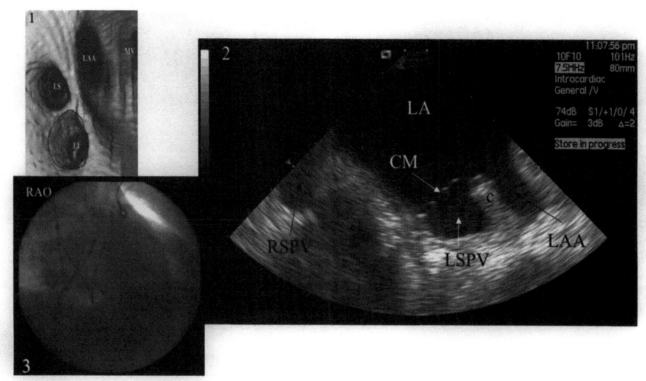

Figure 2.21 *Left superior pulmonary vein and left atrial appendage visualized with MRI (1) and ICE (2). RSPV, right superior pulmonary vein; LSPV, left superior pulmonary vein; LA, left atrium; CM, circular mapping catheter; LAA, left atrial appendage; c, carina between the left superior pulmonary vein and the appendage. Right anterior oblique (RAO) (3) fluoroscopic view showing the position of the intracardiac echo catheter (arrow).*

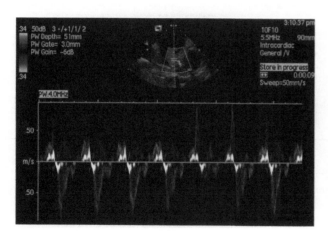

Figure 2.22a *Pulsed-wave Doppler from the right atrial appendage.*

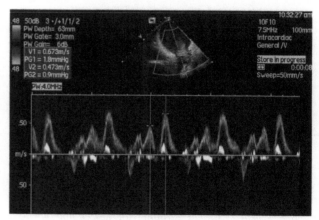

Figure 2.22b *Pulsed-wave Doppler flow from the left superior pulmonary veins.*

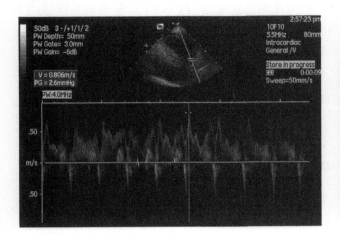

Figure 2.22c *Pulsed-wave Doppler flow from the left superior pulmonary vein immediately after pulmonary vein ablation.*

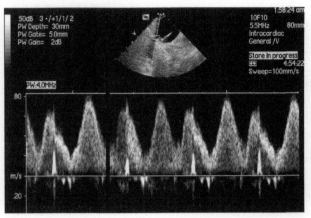

Figure 2.22e *Pulsed-wave Doppler flow from the right inferior pulmonary vein.*

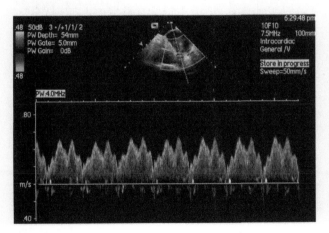

Figure 2.22d *Pulsed-wave Doppler flow from the left inferior pulmonary vein.*

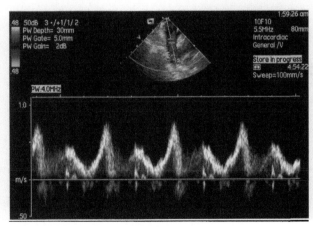

Figure 2.22f *Pulsed-wave Doppler flow from the right superior pulmonary vein.*

REFERENCES

1. Anderson RH, Ho SY, Brecker SJ. Anatomic basis of cross-sectional echocardiography. Heart 2001; 85: 716–20.
2. Yo SY, Anderson RH, Sanchez-Quintana D. Gross structure of the atriums: more than an anatomic curiosity? PACE 2002; 25: 342–50.
3. Anderson RH, Razavi R, Taylor AM. Cardiac anatomy revisited. J Anat 2004; 205: 159–77.
4. Farré J, Anderson RH, Cabrera JA, et al. Fluoroscopic cardiac anatomy for catheter ablation of tachycardia. PACE 2002; 25: 76–94.
5. Waki K, Saito T, Backer AE. Right atrial flutter isthmus revisited: normal anatomy favors nonuniform anisotropic conduction. J Cardiovasc Electrophysiol 2000; 11: 90–4.
6. Ho SY, Sanchez-Quintana D, Cabrera JA, Anderson RH. Anatomy of the left atrium: implications for radiofrequency ablation of atrial fibrillation. J Cardiovasc Electrophysiol 1999; 10: 1525–33.
7. Kato R, Lickfett L, Meininger G, et al. Pulmonary vein anatomy in patients undergoing catheter ablation of atrial fibrillation. Lesson learned by use of magnetic resonance imaging. Circulation 2003; 107: 2004–10.
8. Schwartzman D, Lacomis J, Wigginton WG. Characterization of left atrium and distal pulmonary vein morphology using multidimensional computed tomography. J Am Coll Cardiol 2003; 41: 1349–57.
9. Wittkampf FHM, Vonken EJ, Derksen R, et al. Pulmonary vein ostium geometry. Analysis by magnetic resonance angiography. Circulation 2003; 107: 21–3.
10. Wood MA, Wittkamp M, Henry D, et al. A comparison of pulmonary vein ostial anatomy by computerized tomography, echocardiography, and venography in patients with atrial fibrillation having radiofrequency catheter ablation. Am J Cardiol 2004; 93: 49–53.
11. Marrouche NF, Martin DO, Wazni O, et al. Phased-array intracardiac echocardiography monitoring during pulmonary vein isolation in patients with atrial fibrillation. Impact on outcome and complications. Circulation 2003; 107: 2710–16.
12. Packer DL, Stevens CL, Curley MG, et al. Intracardiac phased-array imaging: methods and initial clinical experience with high resolution, under blood visualization. J Am Coll Cardiol 2002; 39: 509–16.
13. Ren JF, Marchlinski FE, Callans DJ, Herrmann HC. Clinical use of Acunav diagnostic ultrasound catheter imaging during left heart radiofrequency ablation and transcatheter closure procedures. J Am Soc Echocardiogr 2002; 15: 1301–8.
14. Morton JB, Sanders P, Davidson NC, et al. Phased-array intracardiac echocardiography for defining cavotricuspid isthmus anatomy during radiofrequency ablation of typical atrial flutter. J Cardiovasc Electrophysiol 2003; 14: 591–7.
15. Saad EB, Cole CR, Marrouche NF, et al. Use of intracardiac echocardiography for the prediction of chronic pulmonary vein stenosis after ablation of atrial fibrillation. J Cardiovasc Electrophysiol 2002; 13: 986–9.

Chapter 3   The interatrial septum

Samir Kapadia, Atul Verma, Oussama Wazni, and Leonardo Rodriguez

INTRODUCTION

Knowledge of the anatomy of the interatrial septum (IAS) has acquired critical importance in interventional cardiology and electrophysiology. Well-established procedures such as mitral valvuloplasty and pulmonary vein isolation for atrial fibrillation require access to the left atrium via a transseptal approach. Many new procedures such as percutaneous mitral valve repair, aortic valve replacement, and atrial appendage occlusion may also necessitate a transseptal approach. Furthermore, closure of patent foramen ovale and atrial septal defects can now be approached percutaneously in the majority of patients.

DEVELOPMENT OF THE INTERATRIAL SEPTUM

The human interatrial septum is formed during embryonic development by the growth of the septum primum and the septum secundum. The septum primum grows as a crescent from the superior aspect of the atria towards the atrioventricular canal (Figure 3.1). Later, fenestrations appear superiorly in the septum primum to allow communication between the right and left atrium (ostium secundum). A second membrane starts growing from the anterosuperior wall of the atrium, the septum secundum, which covers the ostium secundum (Figure 3.2). The septum primum eventually disappears, leaving a remnant of the membrane covering the fossa ovale (Figure 3.3). This thinner portion can be very mobile and even aneurysmal (>15 mm excursion). In some patients it is referred to as the atrial septal aneurysm. In utero, the septum primum and septum secundum are not fused, allowing blood to shunt from right to left, which is part of the normal fetal circulation. The septum secundum and septum primum fuse in the majority of the population (>60%) after birth, but in approximately one-third of the population the two septa separate from one another transiently when the pressure in the right atrium increases above that of the left atrium: this is called patent foramen ovale (PFO). It is important to note that in these individuals there is no flow of blood between the atria unless the septa are separated by increased right-sided pressure, e.g. with Valsalva or coughing.

IMAGING TECHNIQUES

Echocardiography provides an excellent means of evaluating the interatrial septum. In patients with good imaging windows, transthoracic echocardiography can be used to visualize the IAS. Moderate to large atrial septal defects are easily seen with this technique. Adding color flow mapping allows detection of left to right shunt. When smaller defects are present, using agitated saline during Valsalva increases the detection of intracardiac shunts. Transthoracic echocardiography has important limitations due to resolution and image quality in most patients. It is difficult to see the anatomic details with clarity in most patients because of the anatomic location of the septum behind the sternum and posteriorly. Therefore, in many cases transesophageal echocardiography (TEE) is necessary for a more complete, high-quality evaluation of the IAS. Using TEE, even small PFO can be seen and even small shunts detected by color flow mapping or agitated saline injection. Although TEE provides good images, it is limited by the fact that sedated patients are often not able to perform adequate Valsalva maneuver and hence it may give rise to false-negative results. Furthermore, agitated saline testing from the superior vena cava (SVC) has lower sensitivity than testing done from a lower extremity.

More recently, intracardiac echocardiography (ICE) has provided close, high-resolution images of the IAS.

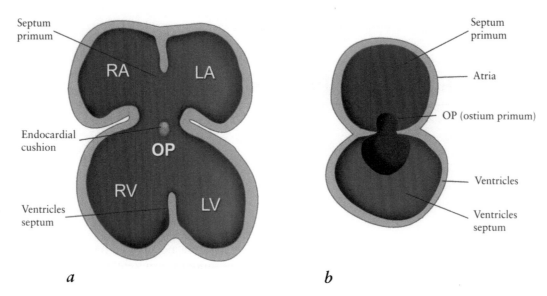

Figure 3.1 *(a) The human interatrial septum is formed during embryonic development by the growth of the septum primum and septum secundum. The septum primum grows as a crescent from the superior aspect of the atria towards the atrioventricular canal. (b) Side view (right).*

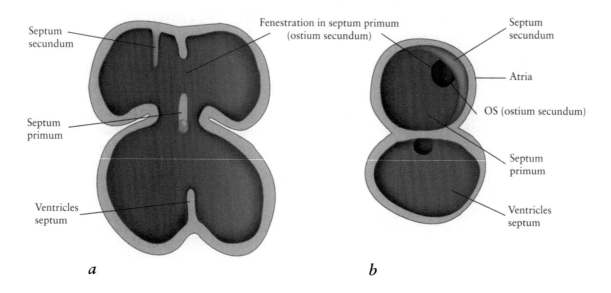

Figure 3.2 *(a) As development progresses, fenestrations appear superiorly in the septum primum to allow communication between the right and left atrium (ostium secundum). A second membrane starts growing from the anterosuperior wall of the atrium, the septum secundum, which covers the ostium secundum. (b) Side view (right).*

Initially, the transducer is kept in the neutral position and rotated in a clockwise direction to see the cardiac structures anterior, to the left and finally to the right and posterior to the inferior vena cava (IVC)–SVC plane. This plane is posteriorly on the right side of the right atrium. When the probe is pointing anteriorly to the right, one can see the tricuspid valve and the

ascending aorta (Figure 3.4). A clockwise rotation from this position allows one to see the interatrial septum. Posterior flexion of the tip creates a gap between the transducer and the septum, allowing visualization of the entire length of the IAS (Figure 3.5). One can adjust the location of the probe in the right atrium to focus either on the upper or lower part of the

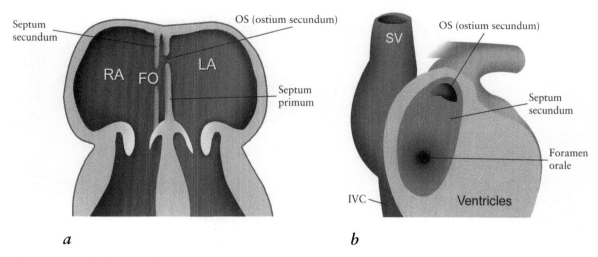

Figure 3.3   *(a) As development further progresses, the septum primum eventually disappears, leaving a remnant of the membrane covering the fossa ovale. (b) Side view (right).*

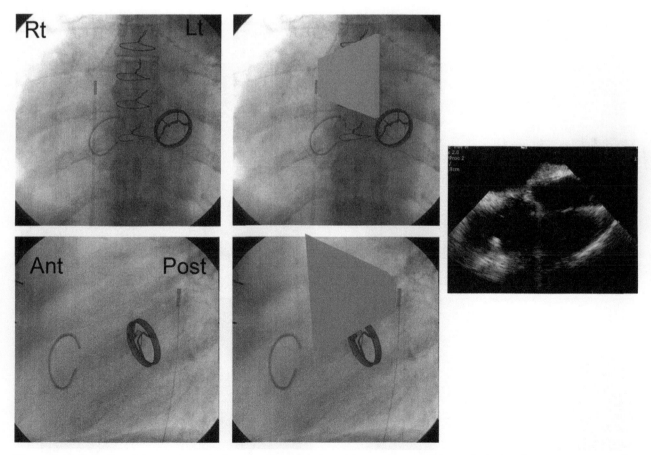

Figure 3.4   *Initially, the transducer is kept in the neutral position and rotated in a clockwise direction to see cardiac structures anterior, to the left and finally to the right and posterior to the IVC–SVC plane. This plane is posteriorly on the right side of the right atrium. When the probe is pointing anteriorly to the right, the tricuspid valve and the ascending aorta can be seen.*

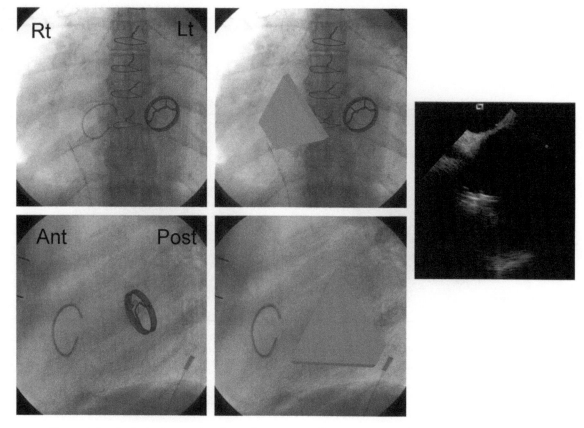

Figure 3.5 *A clockwise rotation from this position allows one to see the entire length of the IAS.*

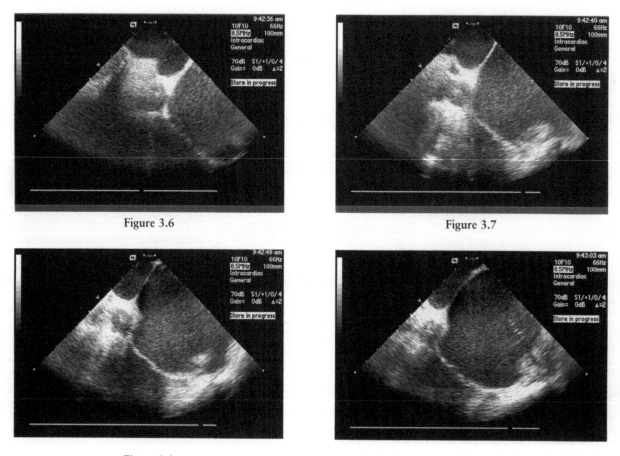

Figure 3.6

Figure 3.7

Figure 3.8

Figure 3.9

Figures 3.6–3.9 *The location of the ICE catheter is advanced from the low right atrium to the mid right atrium showing a normal interatrial septum.*

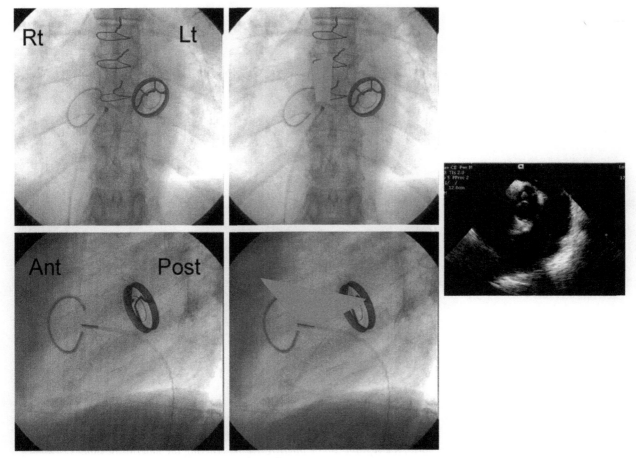

Figure 3.10   *The anteroposterior section of the septum can be visualized by flexing the probe anteriorly and then pointing it to the aorta by counterclockwise rotation. The aortic valve is seen in a cross-sectional view.*

septum. Figures 3.6–3.9 show a normal interatrial septum visualized as the ICE catheter is advanced from the low right atrium to the mid right atrium. The anteroposterior section of the septum can be visualized by flexing the probe anteriorly and then pointing it to the aorta by counterclockwise rotation. The aortic valve is seen in a cross-sectional view (Figure 3.10). Posterior to the aorta, the septum can be interrogated by relaxing the anterior flexion (Figure 3.11).

ABNORMALITIES OF THE INTERATRIAL SEPTUM

In the adult, the interatrial septum can be infiltrated with fat, sparing the fossa ovale, and giving the typical "hourglass" appearance of lipomatous hypertrophy, which should not be confused with tumors such as myxoma (Figure 3.12).

PATENT FORAMEN OVALE AND INTERATRIAL SEPTAL ANEURYSMS

The foramen ovale is an opening between the septum secundum and the septum primum which allows right to left flow in the fetal circulation. After birth there is a functional closure of the foramen ovale due to increasing left atrial pressures. In the majority of people, there is also an anatomic closure in the following months. However, in up to 25% of people the foramen ovale remains patent (PFO). The extent of the opening is variable among individuals, and also depends on the hemodynamic situation. A tiny PFO may become significantly large if the right side pressure increases. In most patients, the communication through the foramen ovale is small and short (Figure 3.13). In other patients, there is more overlapping between the septum primum and the septum secundum, allowing a tunnel-like communication (Figure 3.14). This has practical importance during

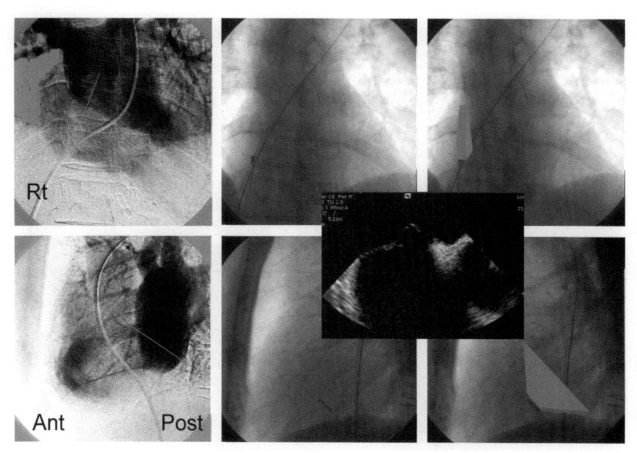

Figure 3.11   *Posterior to the aorta, the septum can be interrogated by relaxing the anterior flexion.*

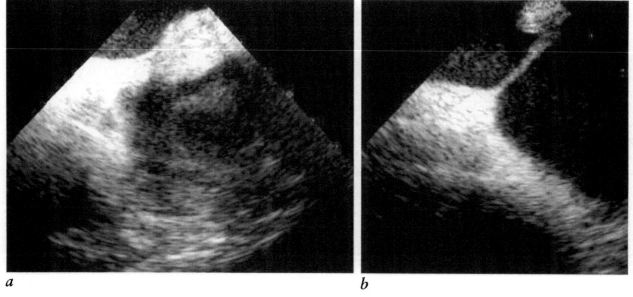

Figure 3.12   *(a) In adults, the interatrial septum can be infiltrated with fat, sparing the fossa ovale, and giving the typical "hourglass" appearance of lipomatous hypertrophy. (b) The lipomatous hypertrophy should not be confused with tumors such as myxoma.*

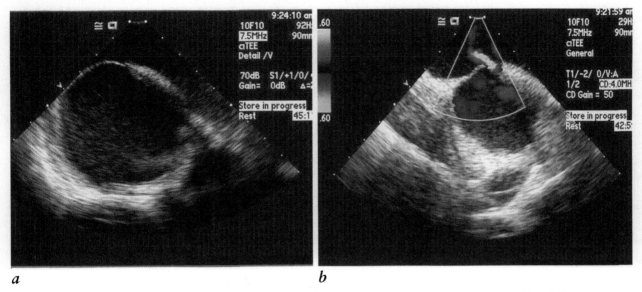

Figure 3.13 *(a, b) In most patients, the communication through the foramen ovale is small and short.*

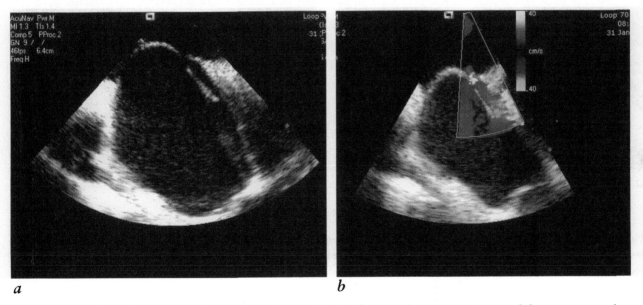

Figure 3.14 *(a, b) In other patients, there is more of an overlapping between the septum primum and the septum secundum, allowing a tunnel-like communication.*

percutaneous closure of a PFO as the device can be entrapped inside the tunnel.

Although in the vast majority of individuals, a PFO is only an incidental finding, large PFO may have clinical relevance. PFO are associated with paradoxical embolism, oxygen desaturation, and decompression illness in divers. Paradoxical embolism occurs when embolic material passing through the RA can, under specific hemodynamic circumstances, cross the PFO and cause cerebral or peripheral embolism. The association between PFO and cryptogenic stroke appears well established, particularly in patients <55 years old. In a meta-analysis, Overell et al found that the odds ratio (OR) for stroke was between 3.0 and 6.0 in patients <55 years old with a PFO. The OR significantly increased if PFO was associated with an interatrial septal aneurysm.

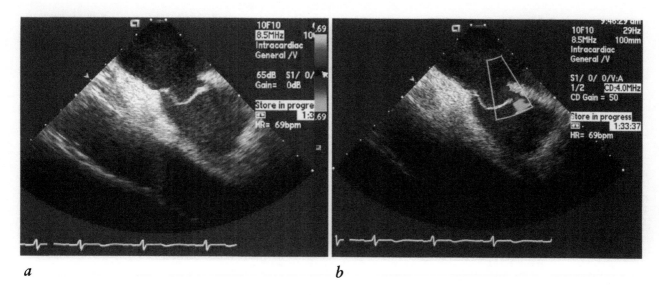

a   b

Figure 3.15

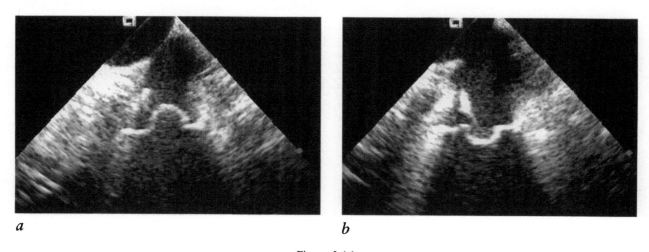

a   b

Figure 3.16

Figures 3.15a,b and 3.16a,b *A typical interatrial septal aneurysm. By echocardiography, the interatrial septal aneurysm is present when the excursion of the septum in total amplitude is >10 mm. Some authors add to this definition, a diameter at the base of aneurysm >15 mm.*

INTERATRIAL SEPTAL ANEURYSM

The septum primum that covers the fossa ovale can be redundant and highly mobile. By echocardiography, the interatrial septal aneurysm (IASA) is present when the excursion of the septum in total amplitude is >10 mm. Some authors add to this definition a diameter at the base of the aneurysm >15 mm. Figures 3.15 and 3.16 show the typical appearance of an interatrial septal aneurysm. A PFO is present in up to 70% of IASA.

Chapter 4 Role of intracardiac echocardiography for ablation of ventricular tachycardia

David J Wilber and Neil Brysiewicz

Intracardiac echocardiography (ICE) has been less commonly employed during catheter ablation of ventricular tachycardia (VT) relative to atrial ablation procedures. Three-dimensional mapping systems in widespread use today render an idealized ventricular geometry that often provides sufficient information for global guidance during catheter mapping. However, such templates do not provide detailed visualization of regions with complex anatomy, or of adjacent structures at risk of injury during energy application. With the availability of deflectable multifrequency phased-array catheters, high-resolution real-time visualization of anatomy, the electrode–tissue interface, and functional properties of the substrate can be routinely obtained during ventricular ablation procedures.[1,2] In many circumstances, particularly for outflow tract tachycardias, ICE provides critical information and online monitoring not readily obtainable by other imaging techniques.

ICE IMAGING DURING RIGHT VENTRICULAR PROCEDURES

The right ventricle can be imaged by positioning the ICE catheter in the low right atrium to visualize the tricuspid valve and the body of the right ventricle (Figure 4.1). The infundibular region and pulmonary valve is best imaged from the right ventricular inflow tract, directing the array superiorly, or from the lateral portion of the outflow tract (Figure 4.2). While ICE imaging is not routinely used in our laboratory during ablation of right ventricular tachycardia, it can provide useful information regarding the presence of anatomic abnormalities suggestive of right ventricular dysplasia.[2,3] In addition, arrhythmogenic foci arising from the pulmonary artery up to several centimeters above the pulmonary valve have been increasingly recognized.[4] Ablation of these tachycardias requires cautious energy titration, and ICE can facilitate accurate localization of the ablation electrode relative to the pulmonary valve, the coronary arteries, and other cardiac structures (Figure 4.3).

ICE IMAGING DURING LEFT VENTRICULAR PROCEDURES

The left ventricle can be imaged by positioning the ICE catheter in the right ventricular inflow tract or deeper in the body of the right ventricle to produce long-axis and short-axis views, identifying normal anatomy and facilitating identification of mapping electrode positions (Figures 4.4 and 4.5). Idiopathic left ventricular tachycardia with a right bundle superior QRS configuration typically involves a re-entrant circuit in the inferior apical septum. The tachycardia is frequently associated with a left ventricular fibromuscular band of variable thickness that extends from the basal septum to the apex or apical lateral wall, often terminating distal to the papillary muscle.[5] This muscular band can be imaged by ICE (Figure 4.6), and provides an anatomic target for ablation when VT cannot be induced by programmed stimulation.[6] In patients with post-infarction VT, it is usually possible to identify the area of infarction on the basis of myocardial thinning and hyperechogenicity associated with fibrosis, as well

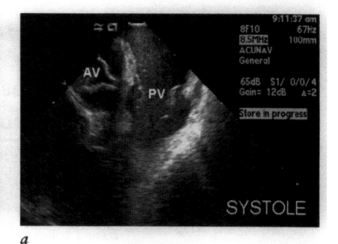

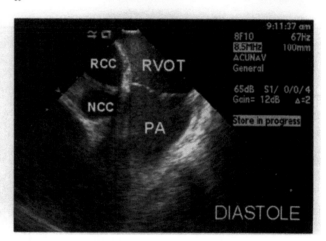

Figure 4.2 *ICE images of the normal right ventricular outflow tract (RVOT), pulmonary valve (PV), and pulmonary artery (PA). Note that the plane of the valve annuli are at 90° to each other. (a) Image in systole, demonstrating both aortic and pulmonary valve leaflets in the open position. (b) Apposition of valve leaflets in diastole. AV = aortic valve; NCC = noncoronary cusp; RCC = right coronary cusp.*

Figure 4.1 *ICE images of the normal right ventricle in 3 different planes. (a) Long-axis view though the body of the right ventricle. (b) Long-axis coronal view. Small arrows indicate a temporary pacing catheter positioned at the right ventricular apical septum. (c) Apical right ventricle, demonstrating a portion of the distal papillary muscle and moderator band (arrow). ant = anterior; inf = inferior; lat = lateral; RA = right atrium, RV = right ventricle; sep = septum; TV = tricuspid valve.*

as abnormal contraction patterns (Figures 4.7 and 4.8). The anatomic border zone between normal myocardium and thinned fibrotic scar can also be identified, providing complementary information relative to scar definition based on electrogram voltage.[7] The border zone is a common exit site and ablation target for the re-entrant circuits of ischemic VT.

One of the most useful roles for ICE is delineation of the complex anatomy of the left ventricular outflow tract during ablation of VT arising from this region.[8,9] Tachycardias may arise near the aortic valve and the coronary artery ostia. Careful definition

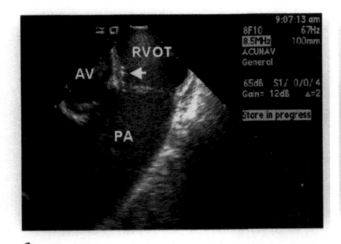

a

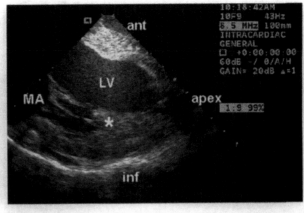

a

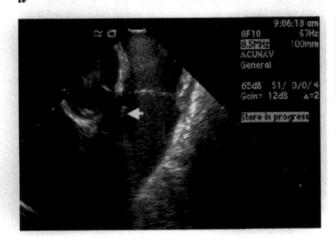

b

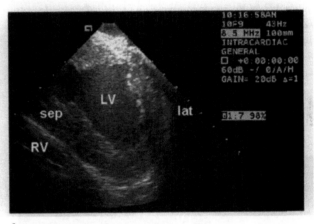

b

Figure 4.3 *(a) Mapping electrode (arrow) positioned at the septal outflow tract, immediately beneath the pulmonary valve. (b) Mapping electrode (arrow) advanced beyond the valve into the pulmonary artery. Abbreviations as in Figure 4.2.*

Figure 4.4 *ICE images of the normal left ventricle (LV). (a) Long-axis view with mitral annulus (MA) to the left and apex to the right. The posterior papillary muscle and associated chordal structures are indicated by an asterisk. (b) Coronal view of the left ventricle. Remaining abbreviations as in previous figures.*

of anatomy, catheter position, and real-time monitoring are extremely useful in facilitating identification of target sites and avoiding arterial injury (Figures 4.9–4.11).

The aortic root can be imaged from either the right atrium or right ventricular outflow tract to produce both short- and long-axis views. Doppler recordings impart additional information regarding coronary flow. A frequent site of origin for outflow tract VT is from the aortic sinuses of Valsalva, where the tachycardia is typically localized to a crescent of ventricular epicardium attached to the base of the aortic leaflets at the arterial–ventricular junction. In our experience with left sinus of Valsalva VT imaged by ICE, the proximal left main coronary artery and the ablation catheter could be imaged in

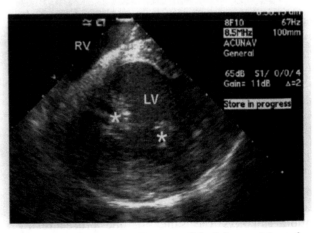

Figure 4.5 *Short-axis ICE image of the left ventricle at the level of the papillary muscles (asterisks), the anteromedial to the left, and the posterolateral to the right.*

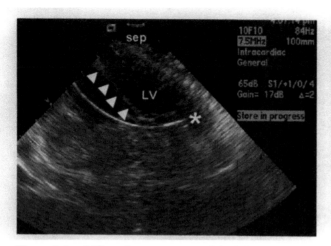

Figure 4.6 *Oblique long-axis view of the left ventricle in a patient with a structurally normal heart and a right bundle, superior axis VT. There is a fibromuscular band approximately 2 mm in diameter traversing the left ventricle from the basal septum toward the inferior apex (arrowheads). There is a mapping catheter with the distal electrode positioned at the apical septum (asterisk).*

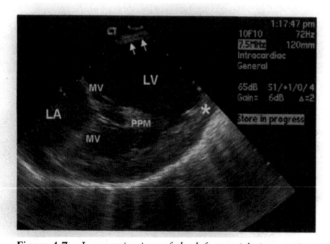

Figure 4.7 *Long-axis view of the left ventricle in a patient with an extensive anterior, septal, and apical scar. Note the normal thickness of the inferior myocardium, with subsequent thinning toward the inferior apex (asterisk). There is marked thinning of the intraventricular septum (arrows). MV = mitral valve; PPM = posterior papillary muscle; other abbreviations as in previous figures.*

all patients. The site of successful ablation and the left coronary ostium are separated by distances ranging from 5–12 mm (see Figures 4.9 and 4.10). Continuous ICE monitoring during energy application enhances the safety of the procedure by assuring catheter stability and monitoring potential adverse effects such as tissue swelling near the coronary ostia during power titration. ICE monitoring may also obviate the need for repeated aortic

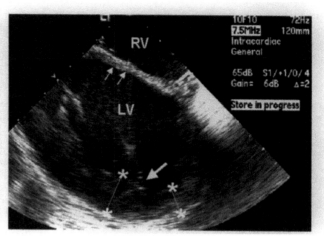

Figure 4.8 *Additional image of the same patient as in Figure 4.7, after slight rotation and advancement of the transducer in the left ventricle. Note again the marked thinning and increased echo density of the intraventricular septum (small arrows), as well as thinning of the apical inferoposterior wall relative to more basal segments (asterisks). During left ventricular mapping of a right bundle superior axis VT, a critical isthmus site defined by electrophysiologic critera was identified at the anatomic inferior scar border, as indicated by the location of the mapping catheter (large arrow). Abbreviations as in previous figures.*

root contrast injections or coronary arteriography. VT may also arise from the left ventricular outflow tract immediately adjacent and beneath the aortic valve in the region of the left fibrous trigone (see Figure 4.11).

OTHER APPLICATIONS

Other applications of ICE for VT ablation include assessment of lesion formation and dimensions, monitoring during energy delivery to assess electrode contact and orientation, and identification and prevention of adverse events during energy delivery. These applications have been explored extensively in experimental models, but have not been routinely applied clinically. In experimental models, tissue swelling and increased echogenicity are frequently detected by ICE following radiofrequency energy delivery.[10] However, consistent and accurate in-vivo assessment of lesion size may require additional enhancements such as myocardial contrast or microbubble injection.[11] Similarly, adverse effects of excessive power delivery in the left ventricle, particularly

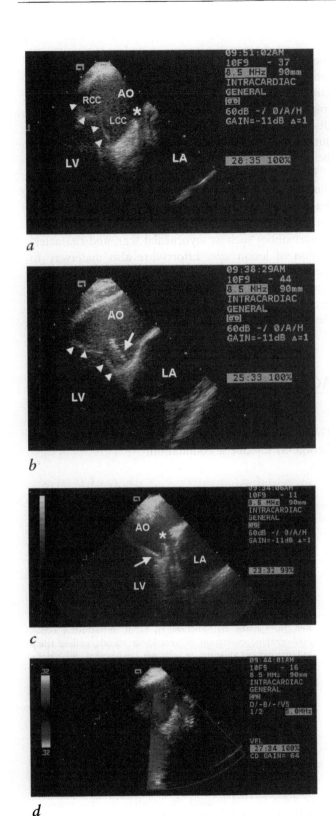

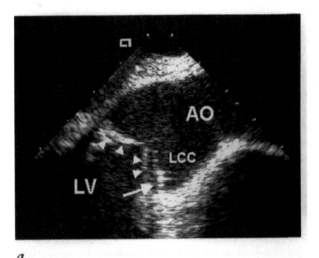

a

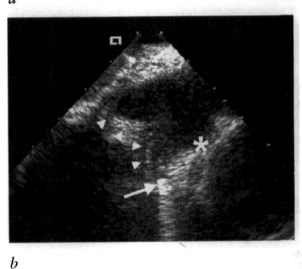

b

Figure 4.10 *ICE images from another patient with left sinus of Valsalva VT. (a) This view of the aortic root demonstrates the ablation catheter (arrow) in the left coronary cusp, but the coronary ostium and the electrode tip are not visualized. (b) With slight rotation of the transducer, both the ostium (asterisk) and the ablation electrode positioned deep in the left cusp (arrow) are simultaneously imaged, separated by approximately 12 mm. Small arrows indicate aortic valve leaflets. As in the previous example, the closest apposition of the ablation electrode to the artery occurs more distally. There is a "flair" artifact immediately below the ablation electrode. Abbreviations as in Figure 4.9.*

Figure 4.9 *ICE images from a patient with VT arising from the left sinus of Valsalva. The aortic root is best viewed in its long axis for this procedure. The aortic valve leaflets in diastolic position are indicated by small arrowheads. (a) Normal anatomy with the left coronary ostium indicated by an asterisk. (b) Position of the mapping catheter (large arrow) a few millimeters above the attachment of the leaflet to the aortoventricular junction. In this view, the left coronary ostium is not imaged. (c) With slight rotation of the*

can be simultaneously imaged. The distance between these two structures is approximately 8 mm. Note that the shortest distance between the mapping electrode and the left coronary artery is not at the ostium, but approximately 1 cm distal to the ostium, where the separation is approximately 5 mm. (d) Color flow Doppler image of the aortic root, demonstrating normal nonturbulent flow through the left main coronary artery (indicated in blue). AO = aorta, LA = left atrium; LCC = left coronary cusp; LV = left ventricle; RCC = right

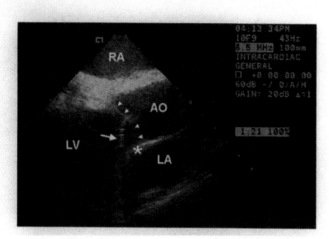

Figure 4.11 *ICE image from another patient with left ventricular outflow tract VT. In this example the earliest site of activation during VT was beneath the aortic valve leaflets (arrowheads). The distal mapping electrode (arrow) is at the anterior mitral annulus adjacent to the left fibrous trigone (asterisk). Abbreviations as in previous figures.*

with the use of large-tip or irrigated-tip catheters, have been characterized by ICE in experimental animals, including steam "pops", and dense showers of microbubbles.[12,13] Such observations provided the current rationale for limits on electrode tip temperature and power delivery for irrigated-tip and large-tip catheters. ICE monitoring may potentially improve the safety of lesion delivery in either ventricle during high-power applications. Whether routine ICE surveillance will improve procedural safety remains to be demonstrated.

Incorporation of new features, such as three-dimensional imaging capability and Doppler tissue tracking,[14] will probably improve the utility of ICE for tachycardia localization, delineation of substrate abnormalities such as myocardial scar, and characterization of lesion size. Efforts are also underway to incorporate anatomic and substrate data from ICE into current three-dimensional mapping systems, providing a more realistic and accurate integration of electrical and structural information.

ACKNOWLEDGMENT

This work was supported in part by a grant from the George M Eisenberg Foundation.

REFERENCES

1. Bruce CJ, Friedman PA. Intracardiac echocardiography. Eur J Echocardiogr 2001; 2(4): 234–44.
2. Jongbloed MR, Bax JJ, van der Burg AE, et al. Radiofrequency catheter ablation of ventricular tachycardia guided by intracardiac echocardiography. Eur J Echocardiogr 2004; 5(1): 34–40.
3. Peters S, Brattstrom A, Gotting B, Trummel M. Value of intracardiac ultrasound in the diagnosis of arrhythmogenic right ventricular dysplasia-cardiomyopathy. Int J Cardiol 2002; 83(2): 111–17.
4. Sekiguchi Y, Aonuma K, Takahasi A, et al. Electrocardiographic and electrophysiologic of ventricular tachycardia originating within the pulmonary artery. J Am Coll Cardiol 2005; 45: 887–95.
5. Thakur R, Klein G, Sivaram C, et al. Anatomic substrate for left ventricular tachycardia. Circulation 1996; 93: 497–501.
6. Merliss AD, Seifert MJ, Collins RF, et al. Catheter ablation of idiopathic left ventricular tachycardia associated with a false tendon. Pacing Clin Electrophysiol 1996; 19: 2144–6.
7. Callans DJ, Ren JF, Michele J, et al. Electroanatomic left ventricular mapping in the porcine model of healed anterior myocardial infarction. Correlation with intracardiac echocardiography and pathological analysis. Circulation 1999, 100: 1744–50.
8. Lamberti F, Calo' L, Pandozi C, et al. Radiofrequency catheter ablation of idiopathic left ventricular outflow tract tachycardia: utility of intracardiac echocardiography. J Cardiovasc Electrophysiol 2001; 12(5): 529–35.
9. Lin AC, Morton JB, Joshi S, et al. Safety and efficacy of catheter ablation of repetitive monomorphic ventricular tachycardia arising from the sinus of Valsalva guided by intracardiac echocardiography. Heart Rhythm 2005; 2: S36.
10. Ren JF, Callans DJ, Michele JJ, et al. Intracardiac echocardiographic evaluation of ventricular mural swelling from radiofrequency ablation in chronic myocardial infarction: irrigated-tip versus standard catheter. J Interv Card Electrophysiol 2001; 5(1): 27–32.
11. Khoury DS, Rao L, Ding C, et al. Localizing and quantifying ablation lesions in the left ventricle by myocardial contrast echocardiography. J Cardiovasc Electrophysiol 2004; 15(9): 1078–87.
12. Callans DJ, Ren JF, Narula N, et al. Effects of linear, irrigated-tip radiofrequency ablation in porcine healed anterior infarction. J Cardiovasc Electrophysiol 2001; 12(9): 1037–42.
13. Wang ZG, Johnson CT, Cooke PA, et al. Comparison of 8-mm tip and irrigated tip catheters for radiofrequency ablation of ventricular myocardium. J Am Coll Cardiol 1999; 33: 140A.
14. Tada H, Toide J, Naito S, et al. Tissue tracking imaging as a new modality for identifying the origin of idiopathic ventricular arrhythmias. Am J Cardiol 2005; 95: 660–4.

Chapter 5   Abnormal anatomy: left atrial structures

Omosalewa O Lalude and Allan L Klein

LEFT ATRIAL APPENDAGE

INTRODUCTION

The left atrial appendage (LAA) is the cul-de-sac region of the left atrium. It is a complex structure that is often multilobed and lined with pectinate ridges, and it varies considerably in size from person to person. The LAA has been recognized as an important part of the cardiac anatomy, owing to its association with thrombus formation and embolic events. This is more so the case with abnormalities of atrial rhythm (fibrillation and flutter) that lead to LAA dysfunction. LAA dysfunction is associated with stagnation of blood flow, which results in a spectrum that ranges from mild spontaneous echo contrast or "smoke", severe spontaneous echo contrast (severe smoke) with or without "sludge", to thrombus formation and thromboembolic disease (Figure 5.1).

ASSESSMENT OF THE LEFT ATRIAL APPENDAGE

Transesophageal echocardiography

Evaluation of LAA structure and function has traditionally been carried out using transesophageal echocardiography (TEE) as a result of its close proximity to the esophageal transducer and the high image resolution provided by this technique. During TEE, the LAA is best assessed at the mid-esophageal level starting at the 0° image plane with the transducer flexed and slightly withdrawn. The transducer is then rotated in increments of 15–30° until the full extent of the appendage is visualized (Figure 5.2). Consequently, multilobed appendages can be thoroughly assessed and the likelihood of mistaking normal structures such as the pectinate ridges as pathology is reduced. It is the

authors' opinion that standard views, e.g. at 0°, 45°, 90°, 120°, or 135°, should be obtained while imaging the LAA to facilitate comparison between subsequent studies.

Transthoracic echocardiography

The utility of transthoracic echocardiography (TTE) in evaluating the LAA has been very limited to date. Recent advancements in transthoracic imaging technology, such as tissue harmonic imaging, have led to improved resolution and better endocardial definition.[1] In addition, tissue Doppler imaging, which now has a significant clinical application in the assessment of systolic and diastolic cardiac function, may also prove to be useful in the assessment of the LAA (Figure 5.3). Visualization of the LAA by TTE can be accomplished in one of three views: the parasternal short axis at the level of the aortic valve, the apical two-chamber, or the apical four-chamber.

Intracardiac echocardiography

The LAA can also be readily imaged by intracardiac echocardiography (ICE). When the ICE catheter is in the mid right atrium at the level of the tricuspid valve (the home view), it is rotated clockwise past the aorta until the LAA comes into view at the level of the mitral annulus[2] (Figure 5.4).

Doppler patterns of the left atrial appendage

The flow patterns of the LAA during TEE are best assessed with pulsed Doppler in the 45–90° image plane, where the Doppler beam is best aligned with

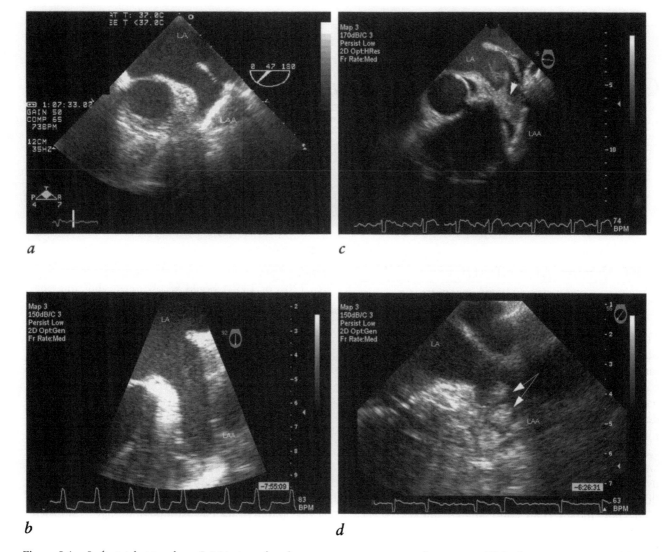

Figure 5.1 *Left atrial appendage (LAA) views that demonstrate spontaneous echo contrast (SEC) due to stagnation of blood flow and rouleau formation: (a) Mild spontaneous echo contrast. (b) Severe spontaneous echo contrast. (c) Arrow points to "sludge" associated with severe spontaneous echo contrast. (d) Double arrow, depicting two echodense structures in the LAA highly suggestive of thrombi in a patient with atrial fibrillation.*

flow. The LAA can also be interrogated by pulsed-wave Doppler during TTE and ICE by placing the sample volume in the LAA cavity at the mid-body level.

Sinus rhythm

In sinus rhythm, the LAA flow pattern is often described as quadriphasic,[3,4] with two forward (emptying) and two backward (filling) flow waves (Figure 5.5a). The first early diastolic forward wave (e) coincides with the early diastolic transmitral and pulmonary venous flows and probably represents passive emptying of the LAA in response to the pressure decline in the left atrium following rapid ventricular filling. It is immediately followed by a diastolic backward filling wave (e'). The second forward emptying wave (a) occurs during atrial systole

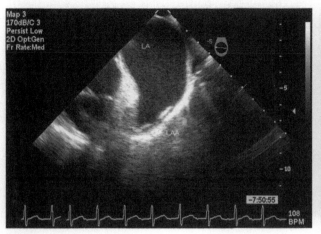

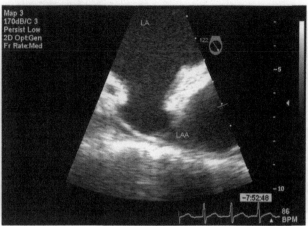

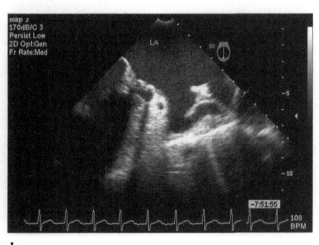

Figure 5.2 *Multiple views of a normal left atrial appendage (LAA) in the same patient: (a) at 0°; (b) at 90°; and (c) at 120°.*

and coincides with the atrial systolic transmitral flow and the atrial reversal wave of pulmonary venous flow.[5] It is followed by the atrial backward filling wave (a′). In contrast to the passive diastolic emptying waves, the atrial systolic waves occur as a result of active LAA contraction and relaxation.

Atrial fibrillation

In atrial fibrillation, the LAA flow assumes a chaotic sawtooth appearance. This represents alternating backward and forward flow signals with varying velocities from beat-to-beat. The LAA velocities are

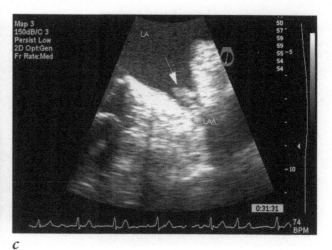

Figure 5.3 *Advancements in technology have led to an improvement in imaging of the left atrial appendage (LAA) by transthoracic echocardiography. (a) Four-chamber view of the LAA enhanced by tissue harmonics. (b) Four-chamber view of the LAA in the same patient with color tissue Doppler imaging. (c) Arrow points to a large protruding thrombus seen during transesophageal echocardiography (TEE) performed later that day in the same patient.*

generally lower than in normal rhythm,[3,6] but they tend to be variable and may occasionally be higher (Figure 5.5b,c). The lower velocities tend to be associated with larger LA/LAA area, mitral valve disease, and LAA containing thrombus/spontaneous echo contrast.

Atrial flutter

In atrial flutter, the LAA flow has a more regular sawtooth appearance than with atrial fibrillation and the velocities tend to be higher[7] (Figure 5.5d). For each emptying/filling cycle, there are several

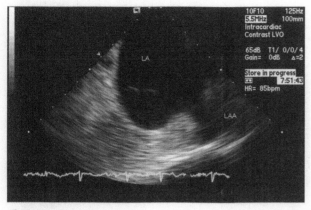

a

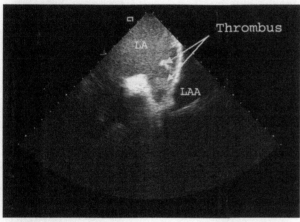

b

Figure 5.4 *Left atrial appendage (LAA) imaging by intracardiac echocardiography (ICE). (a) Normal LAA. (b) Spontaneous echo contrast and LAA thrombi in a 52-year-old man with paroxysmal atrial fibrillation referred for electrical isolation of the pulmonary veins. Transesophageal echocardiography (TEE) was not performed prior to the procedure. This finding led to cancellation of the procedure and continuation of anticoagulation. (Adapted from Jongbloed MR, Bax JJ, van der Wall EE, Schalij MJ. Thrombus in the left atrial appendage detected by intracardiac echocardiography. Int J Cardiovasc Imaging 2004; 20: 113–16, Figure 2. Image courtesy of MR Jongbloed, with permission of Springer Science and Business Media.)*

small non-uniform atrial waves that represent flutter activity.

PULMONARY VEINS

INTRODUCTION

The pulmonary veins return oxygenated blood from the lungs to the left atrium. The right upper and right middle lobar veins usually join together such that the venous drainage from each lung terminates in a superior (upper) pulmonary vein and an inferior (lower) pulmonary vein.[8] These four pulmonary veins then enter the left atrium through orifices in the upper posterior part of the wall. The two left veins may sometimes join and enter the left atrium through a common orifice.[8]

ASSESSMENT OF THE PULMONARY VEINS

Transesophageal echocardiography

Like the LAA, the pulmonary veins (PVs) are usually well visualized by TEE. During TEE, several views are needed for visualization and assessment of the pulmonary veins. At the mid-esophageal level, each vein may be imaged with the sector scan between 0° and 90° with the probe turned to the left or the right.[9] At this level, both inferior (lower) pulmonary veins can be visualized in the transverse image plane at 0° and with slight retraction of the probe superiorly, the superior (upper) veins can be brought into view. The long axis of the left superior/upper pulmonary vein (LUPV) is seen at ~70° in its position next to the LAA (Figure 5.6e), whereas that of right superior/upper pulmonary vein (RUPV) can be seen at 100–120° with the transducer turned to the right (with a forward rotation of 10–20° from the standard bicaval view)[9] (Figure 5.6f). The right superior and inferior PVs can be seen emptying into the left atrium at 45–60° with slight superior retraction and rightward turn of the probe, whereas the left superior and inferior veins can be seen at ~110° with the probe turned to the left[10] (Figure 5.6a–d).

Transthoracic echocardiography

With TTE, the RUPV is the most often visualized. Occasionally, the LUPV is visualized. Compared with

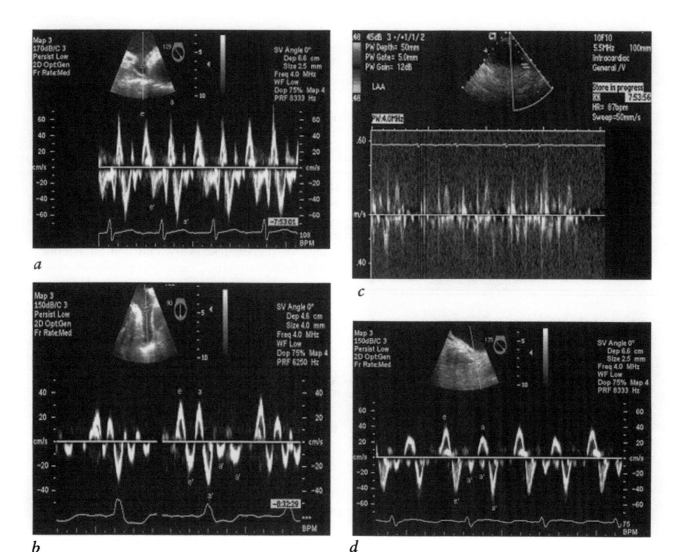

Figure 5.5 *Doppler flow patterns of the left atrial appendage (LAA) by transesophageal echocardiography (TEE) and intracardiac echocardiography (ICE) in normal sinus rhythm (a) atrial fibrillation (b and c) and atrial flutter (d). Note the quadriphasic pattern with two forward emptying waves (e and a) and two backward filling waves (e' and a') by TEE in normal sinus rhythm (a). Note the rapid chaotic and repetitive emptying and filling flow pattern by TEE (b) and ICE (c) in atrial fibrillation. In atrial flutter by TEE (d), there are early emptying and filling waves (e and e') and several smaller non-uniform atrial waves that represent flutter activity.*

TEE and ICE, visualization of the PVs by TTE is very limited. Assessment of the PVs by TTE is, therefore, often limited to interrogation by pulsed-wave Doppler.

Intracardiac echocardiography

The left pulmonary veins can be visualized during ICE by rotating the catheter clockwise from the home view until the left atrium and left PVs are seen (Figure 5.7a). From this position, with further

clockwise rotation and slight superior placement of the catheter, the right PVs should be displayed in cross-section.[2] With further manipulations of the catheter, the long axis of the right PVs may also be displayed (Figure 5.7b,c).

Doppler flow patterns of the pulmonary veins

The pulmonary circulation is in general a low-resistance highly distensible circuit. Flow in the PVs,

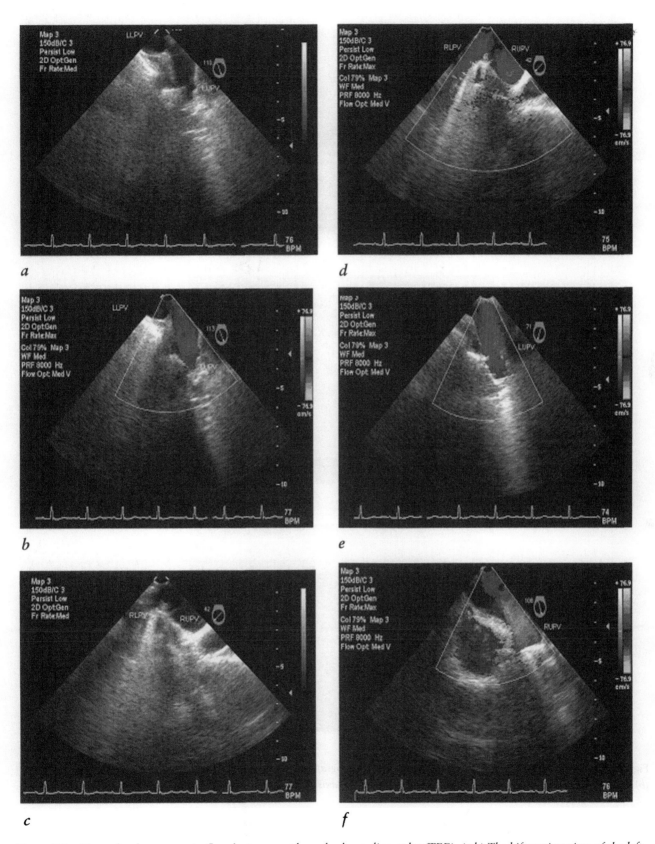

Figure 5.6 *Normal pulmonary vein flow by transesophageal echocardiography (TEE). (a,b) The bifurcation view of the left pulmonary veins in 2D and with color Doppler. (c,d) Bifurcation view of the right pulmonary veins in 2D and with color Doppler. (e) Long-axis view of the left upper pulmonary vein (LUPV). (f) Long-axis view of the right upper pulmonary vein (RUPV).*

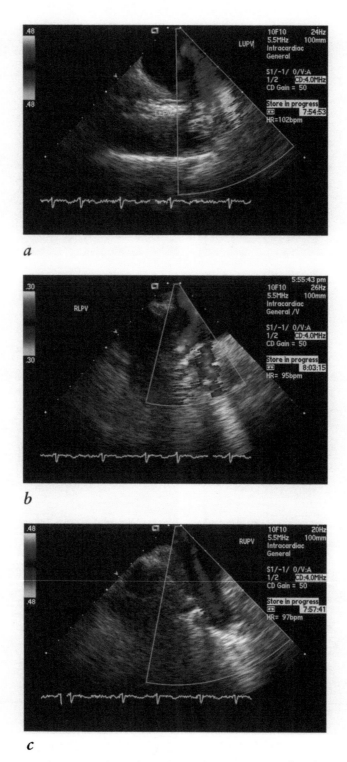

a

b

c

Figure 5.7   *The pulmonary veins by intracardiac echocardiography (ICE). (a) Left pulmonary veins with color Doppler. (b) Right lower pulmonary vein with color Doppler. (c) Long-axis view of the right upper pulmonary vein.*

therefore, tends to be low velocity and should be interrogated by pulsed-wave Doppler with low filter settings.[11]

Sinus rhythm

The normal pulmonary venous flow consists of three waveforms (Figure 5.8). The systolic wave has two components (S1 and S2) and it represents flow into the LA during ventricular systole as a result of atrial relaxation and the suction effect of the heart as it contracts from base to apex. The diastolic waveform (D) is due to a fall in atrial pressure as a result of ventricular filling. The atrial reversal waveform (AR) represents backward flow into the pulmonary veins from atrial contraction in late diastole.[12] During TEE, imaging Doppler interrogation of the PVs is best performed in the long-axis views, where the Doppler beam can be aligned parallel to flow. Normal pulmonary venous low velocity is approximately 40 cm/s. In contrast to TEE, TTE recordings of pulmonary vein flow (PVF) are not as clear, and several studies have investigated ways of improving the quality of these recordings. One study suggested that high-quality recordings of PVF by TTE could be obtained in 90% of patients with current machine technology, sonographer education, and daily practice,[13] whereas another study suggested that contrast injection could enhance the PVF profile.[14]

Atrial fibrillation

In atrial fibrillation, the AR and systolic (S1) waves generated by LA contraction and relaxation, respectively, disappear. In addition, the onset of the S2 wave is delayed and the S2 velocity and systolic fraction are reduced with increased D velocity (Figure 5.9). The velocities of these waveforms are low immediately after conversion to sinus rhythm, but subsequently increase over time.

Pulmonary vein stenosis is a serious potential complication of pulmonary vein isolation (PVI) for the treatment of atrial fibrillation[15–17] (Figure 5.10). Several techniques for PVI have been used, but studies have shown that ablation within the veins is associated with a higher incidence of chronic stenosis than ostial isolation.[16,18,19] Pulmonary vein

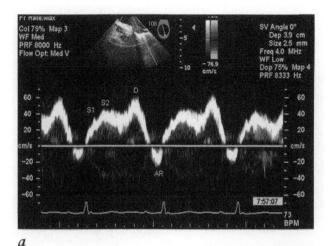

a

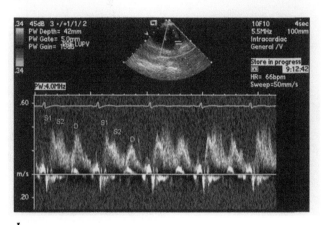

b

Figure 5.8 *Normal pulmonary vein flow pattern: (a) in a 47-year-old woman by transesophageal echocardiography (TEE); (b) in a 60-year-old man by intracardiac echocardiography (ICE). S1 and S2 are the systolic waves, D is the diastolic waveform, and AR is the atrial reversal waveform.*

stenosis is usually treated by stenting through a percutaneous approach (Figure 5.11). The acute increases in flow detected by ICE immediately after PVI have not been shown to predict the development of chronic pulmonary vein stenosis and are thought to be related to inflammation immediately post PVI[20] (Figure 5.12).

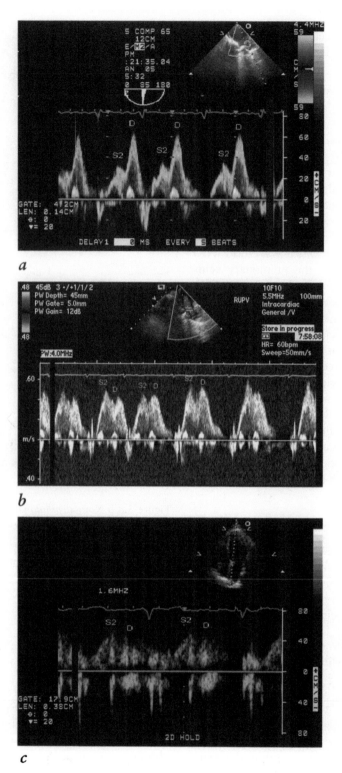

Figure 5.9   *Pulmonary vein flow in atrial fibrillation. Pulsed-wave Doppler obtained on the same day in a 35-year-old man referred for pulmonary vein isolation (PVI): (a) by transesophageal echocardiography (TEE); (b) by intracardiac echocardiography (ICE); and (c) by transthoracic echocardiography (TTE). Note the absence of definite atrial reversal (A) and systolic (S1) waves. Systolic (S2) and diastolic (D) waves are not dependent on atrial activity and are clearly seen. The TTE Doppler recordings were of a poorer quality than the TEE and ICE recordings.*

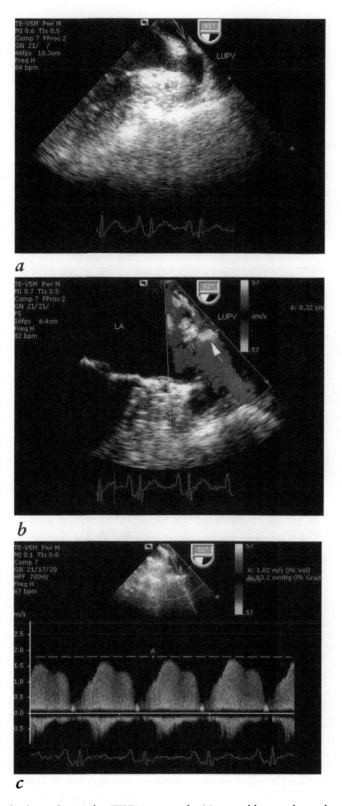

Figure 5.10 *Transesophageal echocardiography (TEE) images of a 44-year-old man who underwent pulmonary vein isolation (PVI) for atrial fibrillation 3 months earlier. A 50% diameter stenosis of the left upper pulmonary vein (LUPV) was noted on a computed tomography (CT) scan. (a) 2D image shows arrow pointing to the stenosis in the LUPV. (b) Color Doppler showing high-velocity flow at the site of the stenosis and formation of an isovelocity convergence zone (arrow) proximal to the obstruction. (c) Pulsed-wave Doppler showing a peak diastolic velocity of ~1.4 m/s (peak systolic velocity was ~1.8 m/s).*

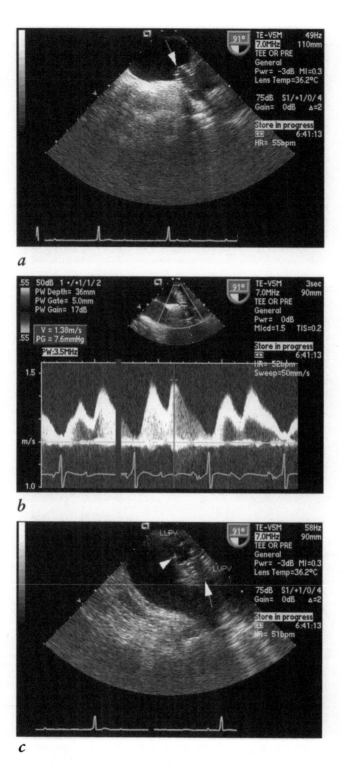

Figure 5.11 *Intraoperative transesophageal echocardiography (TEE) images of a 56-year-old man prior to a MAZE procedure for persistent atrial fibrillation. He underwent two pulmonary vein isolation (PVI) procedures for atrial fibrillation 4 years earlier. Two months after the second procedure, he developed cough and shortness of breath and he underwent balloon angioplasty for pulmonary vein stenosis. The right upper and the left pulmonary veins were subsequently stented for recurrent stenosis: (a) arrow points to a stent in the left upper pulmonary vein (LUPV); (b) pulsed-wave Doppler of the stented LUPV showing an increased diastolic velocity of 1.4 m/s; and (c) stents in the left upper (arrow) and lower (arrowhead) pulmonary veins.*

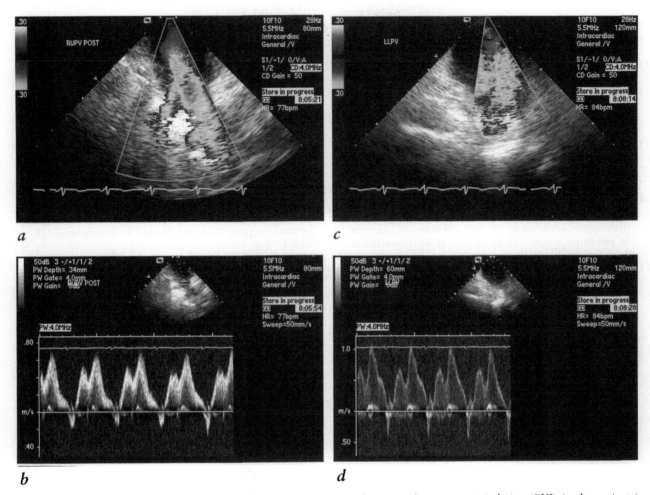

Figure 5.12 *Intracardiac 2D echo and Doppler images immediately post pulmonary vein isolation (PVI) in the patient in Figure 5.9. (a,b) Right upper pulmonary vein (RUPV) is shown by color Doppler. Note the high-velocity flow with color aliasing and the increased diastolic velocity of ~0.8 m/s. (c,d) High-velocity flow is also noted in the left lower pulmonary vein (LLPV). A peak diastolic velocity of 1.0 m/s was noted.*

REFERENCES

1. Ono M, Asanuma T, Tanabe K, et al. Improved visualization of the left atrial appendage by transthoracic 2-dimensional tissue harmonic compared with fundamental echocardiographic imaging. J Am Soc Echocardiogr 1998; 11: 1044–9.

2. Intracardiac echocardiography (ICE) imaging for interventional cardiologists [DVD]. Mountain View: Siemens Medical Solutions USA, Inc; 2004.

3. Jue J, Winslow T, Fazio G, et al. Pulsed Doppler characterization of left atrial appendage flow. J Am Soc Echocardiogr 1993; 6: 237–44.

4. Grimm RA, Stewart WJ, Maloney JD, et al. Impact of electrical cardioversion for atrial fibrillation on left atrial appendage function and spontaneous echo contrast: characterization by simultaneous transesophageal echocardiography. J Am Coll Cardiol 1993; 22: 1359–66.

5. Okamoto M, Hashimoto M, Sueda T, et al. Time interval determination from left atrial appendage ejection flow in patients with mitral stenosis. J Clin Ultrasound 1997; 25: 97–102.

6. Li YH, Lai LP, Shyu KG, et al. Clinical implications of left atrial appendage flow patterns in nonrheumatic atrial fibrillation. Chest 1994; 105: 748–52.

7. Grimm RA, Chandra S, Klein AL, et al. Characterization of left atrial appendage Doppler flow in atrial fibrillation and flutter by Fourier analysis. Am Heart J 1996; 132: 286–96.

8. Malik AB, Vogel SM, Minshall RD, Tiruppathi C. Pulmonary circulation and regulation of fluid balance. In: Murray JF, Nadel JA, eds, Textbook of Respiratory Medicine, 3rd edn (WB Saunders: Philadelphia, 2000) 119–54.

9. Scott DA, Sutton DC. Image planes and standard views. In: Sidebotham D, Merry A, Legget M, eds, Practical Perioperative Transesophageal Echocardiography (Butterworth-Heinemann: New York, 2003) 45–68.

10. Tabata T, Thomas JD, Klein AL. Pulmonary venous flow by Doppler echocardiography: revisited 12 years later. J Am Coll Cardiol 2003; 41: 1243–50.

11. Oh JK, Seward JB, Tajik AJ. The Echo Manual, 2nd edn (Lippincott-Raven: Philadelphia, 1999) 1–5.

12. Sidebotham D, Hussey M. Diastolic dysfunction. In: Sidebotham D, Merry A, Legget M, eds, Practical Perioperative Transesophageal Echocardiography (Butterworth-Heinemann: New York, 2003) 117–30.

13. Jensen JL, Williams FE, Beilby BJ, et al. Feasibility of obtaining pulmonary venous flow velocity in cardiac patients using transthoracic pulsed wave Doppler technique. J Am Soc Echocardiogr 1997; 10: 60–6.

14. Dini FL, Michelassi C, Micheli G, Rovai D. Prognostic value of pulmonary venous flow Doppler signal in left ventricular dysfunction: contribution of the difference in duration of pulmonary venous and mitral flow at atrial contraction. J Am Coll Cardiol 2000; 36: 1295–302.

15. Scanavacca MI, Kajita LJ, Vieira M, Sosa EA. Pulmonary vein stenosis complicating catheter ablation of focal atrial fibrillation. J Cardiovasc Electrophysiol 2000; 11: 677–81.

16. Yu WC, Hsu TL, Tai CT, et al. Acquired pulmonary vein stenosis after radiofrequency catheter ablation of paroxysmal atrial fibrillation. J Cardiovasc Electrophysiol 2001; 12: 887–92.

17. Robbins IM, Colvin EV, Doyle TP, et al. Pulmonary vein stenosis after catheter ablation of atrial fibrillation. Circulation 1998; 98: 1769–75.

18. Lin WS, Prakash VS, Tai CT, et al. Pulmonary vein morphology in patients with paroxysmal atrial fibrillation initiated by ectopic beats originating from the pulmonary veins: implications for catheter ablation. Circulation 2000; 101: 1274–81.

19. Kanagaratnam L, Tomassoni G, Schweikert R, et al. Empirical pulmonary vein isolation in patients with chronic atrial fibrillation using a three-dimensional nonfluoroscopic mapping system: long-term follow-up. Pacing Clin Electrophysiol 2001; 24: 1774–9.

20. Saad EB, Cole CR, Marrouche NF, et al. Use of intracardiac echocardiography for prediction of chronic pulmonary vein stenosis after ablation of atrial fibrillation. J Cardiovasc Electrophysiol 2002; 13: 986–9.

Chapter 6 Intracardiac echocardiography during catheter ablation for atrial fibrillation

Mandeep Bhargava, Robert A Schweikert, Steven Hao, and Andrea Natale

INTRODUCTION

Atrial fibrillation (AF) is the most common sustained arrhythmia. Catheter ablation for AF has been a challenge to interventional electrophysiologists. A major breakthrough in the advancement of catheter-based therapy occurred when it was recognized that atrial fibrillation is triggered by critically timed premature atrial complexes (PACs) from the pulmonary veins[1] (PVs). The pulmonary veins have myocardial sleeves, which have been shown to carry cells with intrinsic automatic activity and the ability to initiate PACs.[2] Initial ablative efforts to suppress these triggers were time-consuming and fraught with limited success and high complication rates, such as pulmonary vein stenosis. The extreme heterogeneity of fiber orientation in and around the pulmonary vein–left atrial (PV–LA) junction may also be responsible for significant electrical disarray which can support re-entry circuits or "rotors" which may sustain AF.[3]

As a result, the concept of pulmonary vein isolation has become an increasingly appealing option. However, the gross and histologic anatomy of the pulmonary veins is more complex than it may appear. Magnetic resonance imaging (MRI) and three-dimensional (3D) computed tomography (CT) have helped begin deciphering the anatomy of the left atrium and the pulmonary veins (Figures 6.1–6.4). The PVs are not just simple cylinders entering a spherical left atrium, rather, they are gradually divergent blood-filled structures which confluence with each other in a complex 3D pattern as they enter the left atrium. Accurate ablation of the PV–LA junction for complete isolation of the triggers from the substrate heavily relies upon real-time imaging, which helps map the asymmetric 3D space, called the "antrum of the pulmonary vein" (Figures 6.5 and 6.6).

In our experience real-time imaging with intracardiac echocardiography (ICE) has been a great help to guide catheter-based pulmonary vein antrum isolation.[4] Over time, we have found ICE to be a complementary tool with fluoroscopy for safe transseptal access, identification of anatomic structures relevant to the ablation, placement and navigation of the circular mapping catheter, titrating energy delivery during

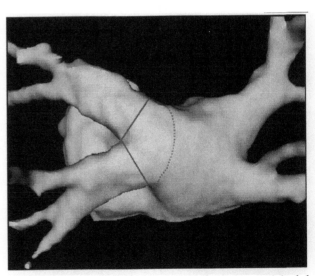

Figure 6.1 *An MRI view of the posterior aspect of the left atrium. It is easy to appreciate the confluence of the two left-sided pulmonary veins (PVs) into a common chamber before they merge into the posterior wall of the left atrium. The tubular portion of the veins is outlined by the green lines and it is usually this level that would probably be visualized as the ostium on a PV angiogram. The border marked by the red lines corresponds to an area far outside the tubular portion, along the seemingly posterior wall of the left atrium. This area corresponds to the "pulmonary vein antrum". Along the roof and the posterior wall of the left atriums, the antrum of the right and left PVs connect with each other.*

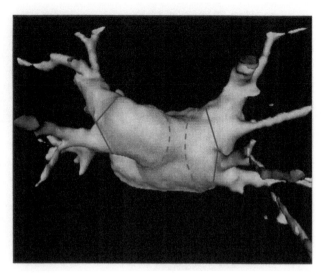

Figure 6.2 *The common confluence of the left pulmonary veins (PVs) is more evident. Even in this example, the antrum of all four pulmonary veins encompasses nearly the entire posterior wall of the left atrium.*

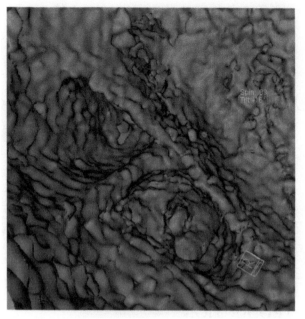

Figure 6.3 *A three-dimensional (3D) reconstruction of the internal anatomy of the left-sided pulmonary veins using 3D CT. The anterior margin of the left pulmonary veins is demarcated by the atrial appendage. Along the posterior, superior, and inferior aspects, the pulmonary veins gradually diverge to enclose a vestibular space which is termed the "pulmonary vein antrum". This knowledge of anatomy is important to define the true "electrically active ostium" of the pulmonary veins.*

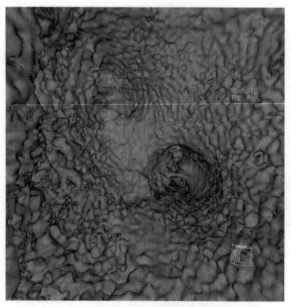

Figure 6.4 *The internal reconstruction of the right pulmonary veins. It is easy to appreciate that the veins gradually diverge in all four directions to merge into the septum anteriorly (the left side of the picture), the roof of the left atrium superiorly, the posterior wall (on the right side of the picture), and along the floor of the left atrium inferiorly. This larger region corresponds to a vestibular space or the "antrum" of the right pulmonary veins.*

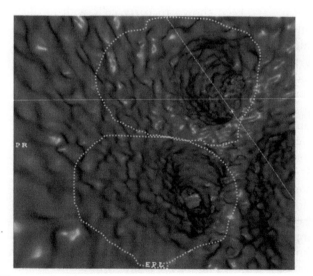

Figure 6.5 *The area that should be ablated along the left PV antra to increase success and reduce the risk of stenosis is depicted by yellow dotted lines. This is far more proximal than the angiographic ostium (shown by the dashed blue lines). Anterior to the left pulmonary veins (PV) is the narrow ridge of tissue separating the PVs from the appendage. At this site, slight deviation posteriorly of the ablation catheter could increase the risk of PV stenosis, and an anterior deviation could result in lesions in the thin wall of the appendage and cause atrial perforation.*

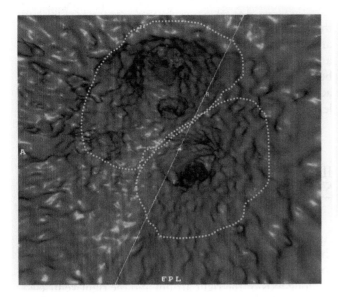

Figure 6.6 *The area that should be ablated around the right PV is depicted by yellow dotted lines. Again, the yellow lines are more proximal than the angiographic ostium (blue circles), and delineate the PV antrum of the right PVs.*

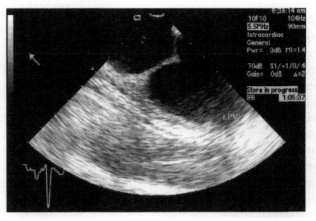

Figure 6.7 *Tenting of the mid portion of the interatrial septum by the Brockenbrough needle inside the transseptal sheath. Note that the left pulmonary veins (LPV) are seen in this plane, signifying that this is the relatively posterior portion of the fossa ovalis.*

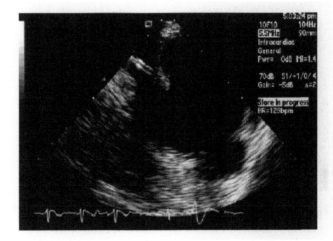

Figure 6.8 *The left superior and inferior pulmonary veins in another patient where the septum is more elastic. In such cases, it is important to visualize the distance from the roof or the posterior wall of the left atrium as the septum could invaginate deep into its cavity.*

ablation, and the early diagnosis of complications. In trying to achieve the best clinical results with catheter ablation for AF at the cost of minimal complications, the critical determinants are to define "where" and "how much" to ablate. In this chapter, we will discuss how ICE has been helpful in our practice in achieving each of these goals.

GUIDANCE OF TRANSSEPTAL PUNCTURE

After the introduction of the catheter in the mid-right atrium, the long-axis view of the tricuspid valve is obtained. This is also called the "home" view. Gentle clockwise motion of the catheter from this point helps in visualizing the long axis of the left atrium and part of the left ventricle, along with the mitral valve and a portion of the aorta. Further clockwise motion brings into view the interatrial septum in the near field. The goal of transseptal puncture in AF ablation is to cross the septum in the posterior region of the fossa ovalis. In the short-axis views of the left atrium, the more anterior portions of the septum are depicted by the views which display the aorta and the left atrial appendage. A puncture along these portions is not only less safe but also directs the catheters more anteriorly towards the mitral annulus, left ventricle, and the left atrial appendage. This can

make the manipulation of catheters difficult for the procedure, as the sheaths would face against the posteriorly placed pulmonary veins.

Further clockwise movement of the catheter from this position displays the more posterior portion of the interatrial septum, which faces the left superior and left inferior veins (Figures 6.7 and 6.8). This plane is our area of choice for crossing the septum to the left side. Further clockwise motion of the transducer displays the posterior wall of the left atrium and then the right pulmonary veins. This plane is more posterior to the ideal transseptal puncture location. ICE allows a safer approach for transseptal puncture even in less experienced hands, to the extent that in our practice we administer heparin even before the transseptal access, to minimize the risk of formation of clots on the sheaths or catheters. ICE allows visualization of the septum, tenting with the needle (Figures 6.7 and 6.8), visualization of adjacent structures, the contrast or saline injection (Figure 6.9) the sheath (Figure 6.10) and the catheters. It is our practice to achieve double transseptal access using Mullen's sheaths, and the second access site is in a similar region (Figure 6.10). Some operators may choose to perform a single transseptal access, advance a guidewire into one of the pulmonary veins, and then withdraw the sheath transiently back into the right atrium. The ablation catheter is then advanced through the same puncture by sliding it along the wire. Once the ablation catheter is in the left atrium, the sheath is pushed back into

the left atrium over the wire. The wire and dilator are subsequently withdrawn. We prefer to perform a double transseptal access to prevent interference between the mapping and ablation catheters and to achieve greater mobility and maneuverability in the left atrium.

IDENTIFICATION OF ANATOMIC STRUCTURES

As described in previous chapters, a quick review of the anatomy is performed in every patient prior to the transseptal puncture. The 'home view' identifies the long axis of the right atrium and the right ventricle along with the tricuspid valve and occasionally a portion of the aorta. Gradual clockwise motion of the probe from this point identifies the long-axis view of the mitral valve, the left atrium and ventricle, and the aorta. This is then followed by the two atrial chambers in their short axis and the left atrial appendage (Figure 6.11). ICE is an adequate tool to confirm the presence of any clot in the left atrial appendage. However, it has not been validated in any prospective trial against the transesophageal echo, which continues to be the gold standard for excluding a left atrial appendage clot. It is also possible to measure the left atrial appendage velocity. In our experience, low left atrial appendage velocities could predict ablation failure[5].

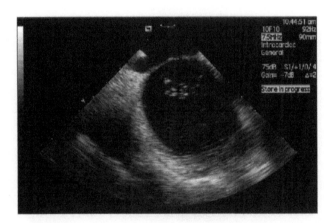

Figure 6.9 *As soon as the needle traverses the septum, injection of saline or contrast can be seen as small bubbles in the left atrial chamber, confirming the position of the tip of the needle in the left atrium. The dilator and the sheath can now be advanced confidently over the needle.*

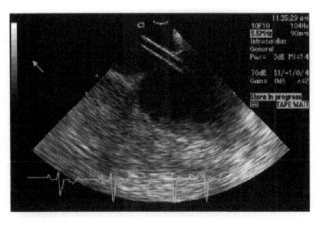

Figure 6.10 *The transseptal sheath across the mid-portion of the interatrial septum.*

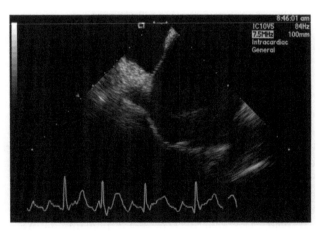

Figure 6.11 *A view of the tail-like extension of the left atrium, the left atrial appendage. The thin portion of the interatrial septum in the region of the fossa ovalis can be seen at the top of the picture and has a sharp demarcation with the relatively thicker portion higher up. This is a relatively anterior portion of the septum and not the most preferred site of transseptal access for a pulmonary vein (PV) antrum isolation procedure.*

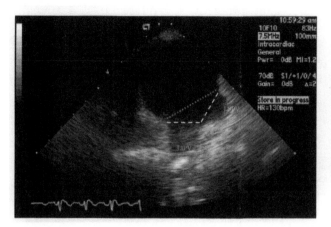

Figure 6.12   *A short-axis view of the left atrium, along with a long-axis view of the left superior and the left inferior pulmonary veins. Most often, both veins can be seen in their long axis in the same view. The first to appear is the left superior pulmonary vein, which lies relatively horizontal in the picture and is seen at 4 o'clock in this figure. The left inferior pulmonary vein appears somewhat vertically and appears at 6 o'clock. The white dotted line corresponds to the ostium of the tubular portions of the pulmonary veins, but the red stripes correspond to the wider area, which corresponds to the opening of the pulmonary vein (PV) antrum. The two left pulmonary veins almost always form a small common confluence before entering the left atrium. This reflects the posterior extension of the PV antrum (demarcated between the red and white lines). Isolation of the veins at a more proximal level is essential to achieve maximum efficacy from catheter ablation. The veins can be easily differentiated from the atrial appendage by observing pulse Doppler flows in the pulmonary veins, which show a characteristic biphasic flow pattern.*

With further clockwise rotation, one can visualize a short-axis view of the left atrium with the left pulmonary veins on the bottom right of the screen (Figures 6.12 and 6.13). The left superior vein is seen first and appears higher up in relation to the left inferior vein, which is visible on further clockwise rotation of the ICE catheter. Most often, both the left-sided pulmonary veins can be seen along their long axis in the same view; but sometimes their orientation may be such that they can be viewed only one at a time. The superior pulmonary vein has a relatively more horizontal appearance on the screen and the inferior vein is relatively more vertical. The inferior vein is also related to the aorta, which can be visualized along its long axis with gentle manipulation of the catheter. Color Doppler (Figure 6.14) and pulse wave Doppler (Figure 6.15) can be used to characterize and confirm flow across the pulmonary veins.

After identifying the anatomy of the left pulmonary veins, further clockwise motion of the transducer

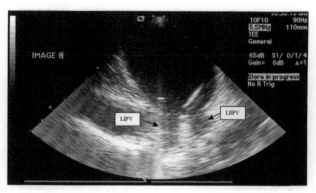

Figure 6.13   *An example of a patient where the left-sided pulmonary veins (PVs) are relatively more tubular and only have a small common antrum as they enter the left atrium. The PVs enter the atrium through a more discretely defined ostia, and are depicted in green and yellow for the left superior pulmonary vein (LSPV) and the left inferior pulmonary vein (LIPV), respectively. This finding is unusual and is seen in no more than 5–10% of the patients. Even in such a case, the circular catheter is moved out to the continuous line representing the short posterior extension of the left "antrum."*

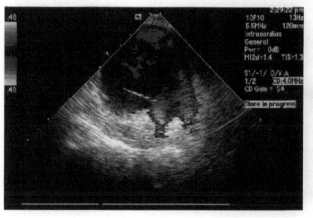

Figure 6.14   *The color Doppler picture of flow across the left superior and left inferior pulmonary veins. Red defines blood moving in the direction of the transducer.*

gives a view of the right superior and inferior pulmonary veins (Figure 6.16). This view, which is also called the "owl-eye" view, shows a cross-sectional view of the ostia of the two right-sided pulmonary veins. The right superior PV is seen above and the right inferior of the PV and color Doppler and pulsed-wave Doppler can be used to confirm flow typical of the pulmonary veins (Figure 6.17). A longitudinal view of the right-sided veins can also be obtained. For this view, the transducer is first rotated approximately 180° from the home view against the direction of the interatrial septum. Then it is retroflexed by about

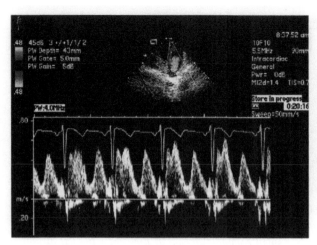

Figure 6.15 *Pulse Doppler flow through the left superior pulmonary vein. Normal systolic and diastolic pattern of flow can be demonstrated and confirms pulmonary venous flow. We tried to compare the pre- and post-ablation flow velocities to see if changes with ablation are predictors for the occurrence of stenosis, but no correlation could be demonstrated.[6] However, other groups have shown that velocities above 1.5 m/s (not seen in our series) are associated with an increased risk of chronic PV stenosis.[7]*

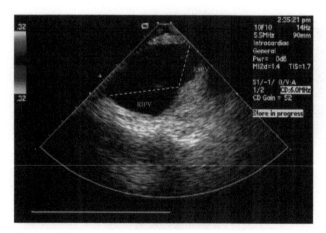

Figure 6.16 *A short-axis view of the right superior pulmonary vein (RSPV) and the right inferior pulmonary vein (RIPV). The respective ostia of the two veins are depicted by dashed white lines.*

45° or more to obtain a longitudinal view of the right inferior pulmonary vein (Figure 6.18). In contrast to the other three pulmonary veins, this vein usually has the shortest main stem and branches very early in its course. The short tubular portion of this vein is inferior and posterior to the right superior pulmonary vein and has less of a funnel-shaped portion than the other pulmonary veins.

It is unusual for both right pulmonary veins to be visualized in their longitudinal axis in the same frame. It usually requires further clockwise motion of the

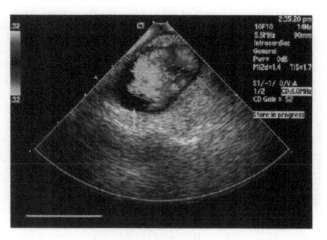

Figure 6.17 *The color Doppler flow through the right superior (green arrow) and the right inferior (yellow arrow) pulmonary veins. This, in conjunction with pulsed-wave Doppler, can be used to confirm the ostium and the flow velocity inside the pulmonary veins.*

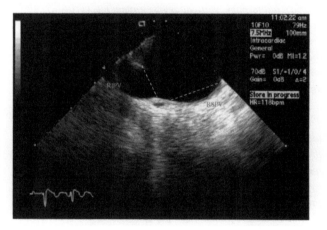

Figure 6.18 *A long-axis view of the right inferior pulmonary vein (RIPV), lying just next to the interatrial septum, the thin portion of which is barely visible in the near field of this view. The cross section of the right superior pulmonary vein (RSPV) is also visible in this view. It is unusual for the long axis of both the right-sided veins to be visible in the same view. The two respective ostia are shown by broken white lines and the area between the two lines depicts the carina or the junction between the two pulmonary veins. This carina is usually thicker and more prominent on the right side when compared to that on the left side. The RIPV usually has a short tubular segment and branches very early in comparison with the other veins.*

transducer from the position showing the long axis of the right inferior PV to visualize the long-axis view of the right superior PV (Figure 6.19). The proximity of the right superior pulmonary vein to the right pulmonary artery can be appreciated in this view, as the latter is seen just behind the vein (Figure 6.20). This relationship can help differentiate

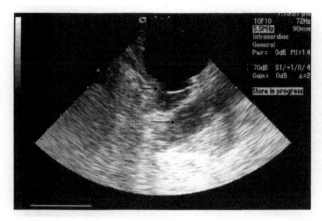

Figure 6.19 *Further clockwise motion of the transducer from the previous view shows the long axis of the right superior pulmonary vein (RSPV). As the two right-sided veins are not usually seen on the same view, the RSPV can be differentiated by its vertical orientation on this view, the relationship with the right pulmonary artery (RPA), which is seen behind the RSPV in its long axis, and also by the fact that it has a longer tubular portion with a proximal funnel-shaped pattern (better appreciated in Figure 6.20).*

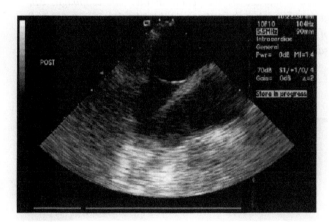

Figure 6.20 *The long-axis view of the right superior pulmonary artery (RSPV). The left atrium lies in the near field of the picture and the right pulmonary artery is seen with a horizontal orientation in the far field. The RSPV shows a more prominent divergence in this view as it enters the left atrium. The circular mapping catheter is seen at the ostium of the right superior pulmonary vein.*

the right superior PV from the right inferior PV. The right pulmonary veins form a vestibule, which extends both anteriorly and posteriorly and needs to be completely isolated to maximize success. The left and right veins can be seen in close proximity to each other (Figure 6.21). This shows how the two pulmonary venous antra merge into each other along the posterior wall.

Our strategy for ablation for atrial fibrillation also includes isolation of the superior vena cava (SVC)

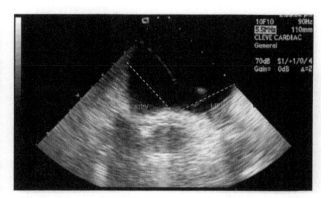

Figure 6.21 *An example showing the antrum of the right inferior pulmonary vein (RIPV) and left inferior pulmonary vein (LIPV), respectively, in their cross-sectional view. The two antra are delineated by dashed white lines. Posteriorly, there is a very narrow rim of tissue in between these two antra (as marked by the red arrows), which again indicates that the posterior wall is often just the confluence of the posterior extensions of the antrum of the right and left PVs.*

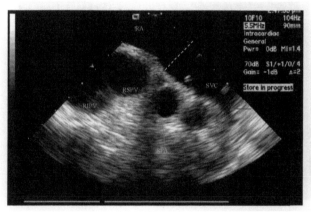

Figure 6.22 *A long-axis view of the superior vena cava–right atrial (SVC–RA) junction. The right superior pulmonary vein (RSPV) and the right inferior pulmonary vein (RIPV) are seen on the left of the picture and the right atrium on the top. The long axis of the SVC courses on the right of this view. The two branches of the right pulmonary artery (RPA) can be seen above the pulmonary veins, as marked by the green arrows, and the azygos vein can be seen arching over the pulmonary arteries (as marked by the red arrow). Often, the right main pulmonary artery can be seen instead of the two branches, and just below the pulmonary arteries is a small triangular area along the septal border of the SVC. This marks the junction of the SVC and the RA and is depicted by the white dashed line.*

in all patients who show evidence of pulmonary vein-like potentials along the superior vena cava–right atrial (SVC–RA) junction. ICE is extremely useful to define the SVC–RA junction, as can be seen in Figure 6.22.

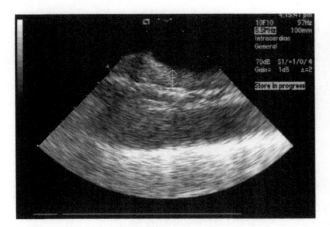

Figure 6.23 *The esophagus on ICE in relation to the posterior wall of the left atrium (LA), as depicted by the red arrow. The yellow arrow shows the distance between the endocardium of the LA and the outer wall of the esophagus.*

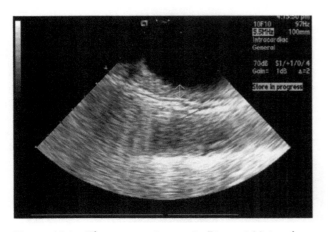

Figure 6.24 *The same patient as in Figure 6.23 in whom visualization of the esophagus has been enhanced by administration of a small amount of carbonated beverage.*

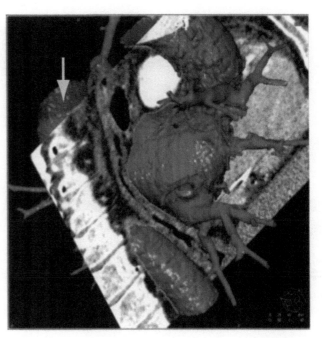

Figure 6.25 *A sagittal section of a CT scan of the left atrium and its relation to the esophagus. The esophageal lumen is marked by the yellow arrow. The esophagus can be seen coursing along the entire length of the posterior wall of the left atrium (LA). Note the lack of any significant adventitious tissue separating the two structures.*

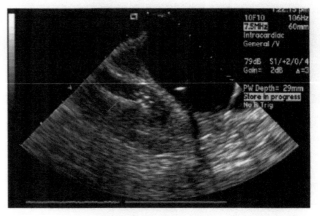

Figure 6.26 *An example of the esophagus (as depicted by the red arrow) in relation to the left pulmonary veins.*

Another important structure that can be visualized by ICE is the esophagus (Figure 6.23). The esophagus has a variable relationship to the left and right pulmonary veins and the posterior wall (Figures 6.25–6.28). Visualization of the esophagus can be enhanced by the ingestion of carbonated beverage (Figure 6.24). The thickness of the atrial wall adjacent to the esophagus varies from 1.9 mm to 4.2 mm, with an average thickness of 2.8 ± 0.9 mm. Sometimes the position may vary in the same patient during different times of the study. Other groups have reported shifting of the anatomic relationship between the esophagus and the left atrium. This, however, has been seen only after the administration of barium paste and has not been confirmed in our experience.

Identification of the esophageal relationship can prevent occurrence of atrio-esophageal fistulas, by either controlling or avoiding energy delivery during ablation in this region. In our experience, energy application by monitoring for microbubbles has been very useful and has not resulted in this complication in over 2000 procedures.

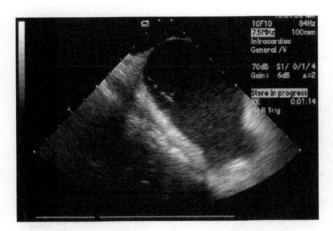

Figure 6.27 *Another patient in whom the esophagus can be seen in relation to the left pulmonary veins.*

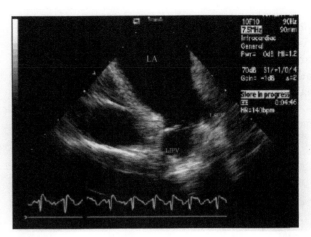

a

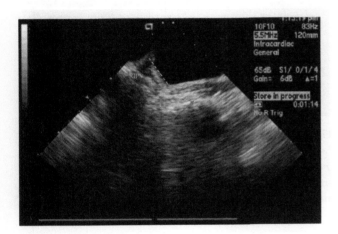

Figure 6.28 *The esophagus in relation to the right inferior pulmonary vein (RIPV). The ostium of the RIPV is shown by the dashed white line and the esophagus is marked by the red arrow.*

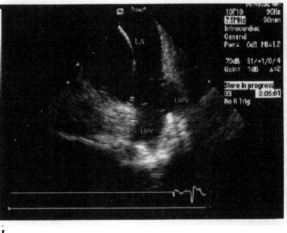

b

Figure 6.29 *(a) An example of a patient with a common ostium of the left pulmonary veins. The left superior pulmonary vein (LSPV) and the left inferior pulmonary vein (LIPV) merge into a common opening, which measures about 1 cm in depth and then opens into the left atrium (LA) through a large, clearly demarcated common ostium. The circular mapping catheter is seen at the ostium of the tubular portion of the LIPV as shown by the red arrow. The isolation of the pulmonary vein at this level would lead to incomplete pulmonary venous antral–left atrial disconnection and would also increase the risk of pulmonary venous stenosis. Placement of the mapping catheter at this level is helpful only for ablation of the anterior segments of the left pulmonary veins (as discussed later in the chapter). (b) For completion of the isolation of the antrum, the circular mapping catheter has to be moved more proximally, as indicated by the green arrow. The ablation catheter tip can also visualized by ICE, as seen in this frame.*

ANATOMIC VARIATIONS

The anatomic variations of the interatrial septum and the appendage have been described in other chapters of this book. There can sometimes be interesting variations in the anatomy of the pulmonary veins. These are rare and are easier to pick up on the CT/MRI or ICE images rather than on the PV angiogram.

Based on CT and MRI findings, about 10–15% of patients have an easily appreciable common ostium on the left PVs (Figure 6.29a and 6.29b). The left superior and inferior PVs clearly confluence into this common chamber, which measures 1–2 cm in length, and, in turn, drains into the left atrium

through a common opening. This can be especially hard to appreciate on the pulmonary venous angiogram, because the contrast dilutes as it moves out into the common chamber. A short common confluence of the left pulmonary veins is not unusual on ICE, and, as mentioned before, could be present in nearly 85–90% of patients. It is important to appreciate this variation in PV anatomy, as the circular mapping catheter would need to be placed much more proximally to isolate the antrum (Figure 6.29b). A common

ostium of the right PVs is found in less than 25% of the patients and is also of a much shorter length (Figure 6.30).

At times, there may be more than two pulmonary veins on one side. In our experience, this is observed in less than 1% of the patients and is more common in the right PVs (Figure 6.31). The right middle pulmonary vein is almost always a tributary of the right superior pulmonary vein but rarely drains through a separate ostium into the left atrium. It is important to appreciate

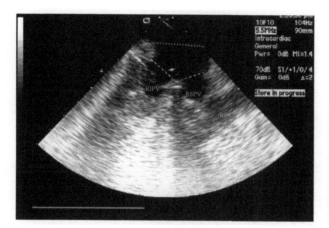

Figure 6.30 *An example of a common ostium of the right pulmonary veins. The longitudinal axis of both the right superior and the right inferior pulmonary veins are seen in the same view (RSPV and RIPV, respectively) and the right pulmonary artery (RPA) is seen posterior to the RSPV. The dashed white lines correspond to the ostium of the tubular portion of the two pulmonary veins. The dotted red line defines the true antrum, which is the level at which isolation has to be achieved to maximize the chances of cure of atrial fibrillation.*

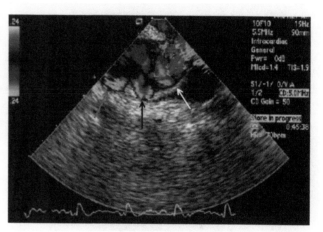

Figure 6.31 *An example of a patient with three separate ostia on the right side. This is a short-axis view that shows a cross-sectional image of the three ostia of the right inferior (red arrow), right middle (black arrow), and the right superior (white arrow) pulmonary veins.*

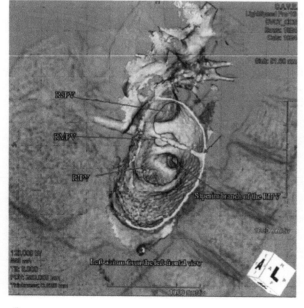

a

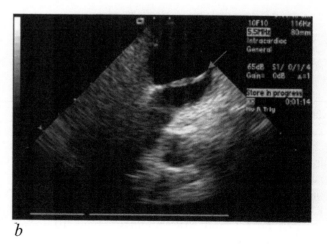

b

Figure 6.32 *(a,b) A very rare abnormality which has not been described. The CT scan and the long-axis view of the right superior pulmonary vein (RSPV) on ICE show a false tendon in the left atrium, which has one limb connecting close to the os of the right superior pulmonary vein. The arrow shows the tendon traversing across the opening of the RSPV. RMPV = right middle pulmonary vein; RIPV = right inferior pulmonary vein.*

this variant, as all three pulmonary veins need to be isolated. By ICE, the right PV antrum is treated as a large vestibule that includes all the PVs. Another rare abnormality is shown in Figure 6.32a and b. This reflects a false tendon that was noted in the left atrium.

PLACEMENT OF THE CIRCULAR MAPPING CATHETER

The next part of the procedure in which ICE is particularly useful is the placement of the circular mapping catheter. The mapping and the ablation catheters, with their electrodes, can be visualized when advanced into the left atrial chamber. Combining fluoroscopy and ICE, the mapping catheter is placed in various positions along the whole circumference of the left and right pulmonary vein antrum. The circular catheter becomes a guide for the ablation catheter when applying radiofrequency (RF) lesions to isolate the pulmonary vein antrum. Unless the size of the pulmonary veins is extremely small, we almost always use a standard 10-pole 20 mm diameter circular mapping catheter. True antrum isolation requires abolition of all PV potentials that extend to the PV antrum proximal to the tube-like portion of the PV.

Figures 6.33 through 6.35 are examples showing the intracardiac recordings from the circular mapping catheter during the various stages of the procedure. These electrograms are recorded from the anterior (Figures 6.33, 6.34a and b) and the posterior (Figures 6.35a and b) segments of the left superior pulmonary vein, before and after delivery of RF energy. This example highlights the importance of differentiating between the electrical signals from the pulmonary

venous sleeves, the atrial tissue and the atrial appendage.

Since ICE can provide continuous geometric information on the cardiac structures, its use in addition to fluoroscopic and electrophysiologic mapping increases the accuracy of catheter placement, provides real-time visualization of the catheters in relation to the complex geometry of this anatomic region, and has the potential advantage of limiting the fluoroscopic exposure for both the patient and the operators. ICE also helps in defining the ostium of the pulmonary venous antrum. The example shown in Figures 6.36a and 6.36f demonstrate how the definition of the

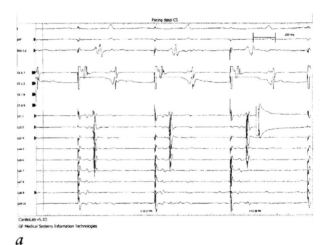

a

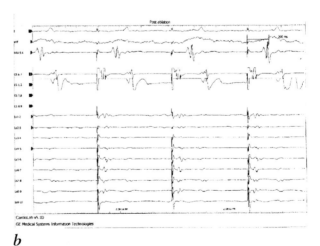

b

Figure 6.34 *(a,b) Examples of ICE recordings from the left superior pulmonary vein (LSPV) in the same patient after cardioversion. (a) The recordings during pacing of the distal coronary sinus (CS). This helps to differentiate between the low-frequency, low-amplitude atrial signals and the high-frequency pulmonary vein (PV) potentials. (b) After ablation, the high-frequency PV potentials are no longer seen as a result of the entrance block within the PV, but the low-frequency atrial signals persist.*

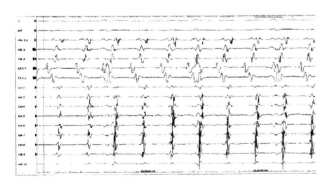

Figure 6.33 *The intracardiac recordings from a patient with recurrent atrial fibrillation and atrial flutter who presented for pulmonary vein antrum isolation. The patient had atrial flutter at presentation and the recordings on the circular mapping catheter (Ls3-4 to Ls9-10) demonstrate high-frequency pulmonary vein potentials.*

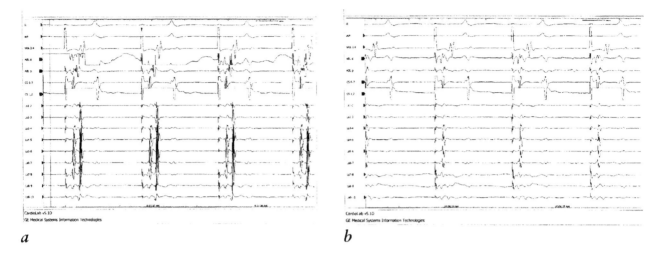

a　　　　　　　　　　　　　　　　　　*b*

Figures 6.35 *(a,b) A similar example to Figure 6.34 in another patient. The electrograms are displayed during distal coronary sinus (CS) pacing before (a) and after (b) the ablation. In this example, the mapping catheter is close to the border of the left atrial appendage. Hence, in addition to the atrial electrogram and the pulmonary vein (PV) potentials, one can appreciate the far-field recording from the left atrial (LA) appendage. After the ablation, the PV potentials have disappeared but the atrial and left atrial appendage electrograms persist.*

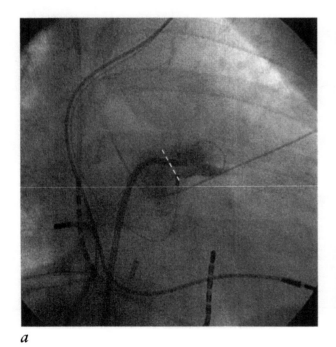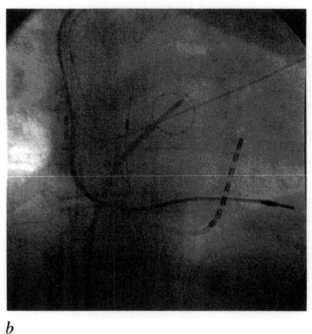

a　　　　　　　　　　　　　　　　　　*b*

Figure 6.36a *Figures 6.36a–6.36f show a demonstration of the difference between the definitions of the ostium by pulmonary vein angiogram versus ICE. An example of a pulmonary vein angiogram of the left superior pulmonary vein in the right anterior oblique (RAO) view. The dashed white line shows the ostium as would be defined by the venogram.*

Figure 6.36b *The placement of the circular mapping catheter at the ostium of the pulmonary vein, as defined by the venogram in the same view.*

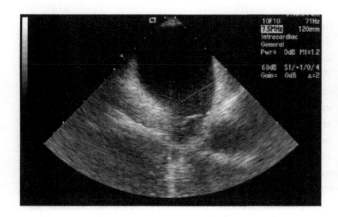

c

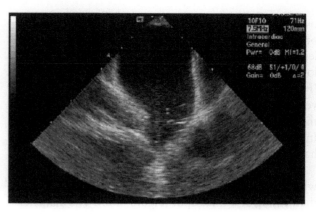

d

Figure 6.36c *The simultaneous position of the circular mapping catheter on ICE when it was placed at the ostium, as defined by the pulmonary vein angiogram (yellow arrow). This would correspond to the ostium of the tubular portion of the pulmonary vein, and hence would be the desired position to guide the ablation along the anterior segments of the left superior pulmonary vein antrum. However, angiography would miss the more proximal funnel-shaped portion of the pulmonary vein antrum along the other three aspects of the vein. This area would correspond to the region close to the dashed red line.*

Figure 6.36d *The more proximal placement of the circular mapping catheter guided by ICE.*

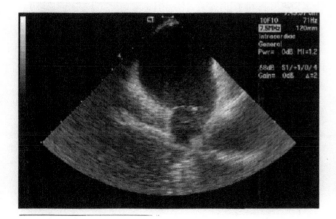

e

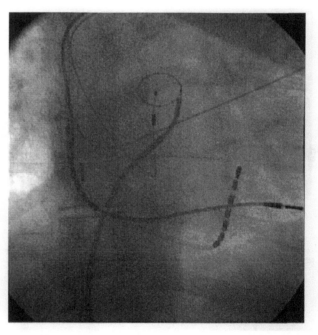

f

Figure 6.36e *In the same patient, the circular mapping catheter is moved to the lower portion of this large common left PV antrum. This corresponds to the inferior portion of the dotted red line in Figure 6.36c. Isolation at this level is likely to be associated with a higher rate of cure and a lower risk of pulmonary vein stenosis.*

Figure 6.36f *The corresponding fluoroscopic picture of the circular mapping catheter when placed in the left superior pulmonary vein, as shown in Figure 6.36d. Note the difference in position in comparison to the placement by the PV angiogram in Figure 6.36b.*

ostium on ICE is much more proximal to that defined on a PV angiogram. This helps in delivering the lesions proximally, resulting in higher efficacy and lower risk of complications. The subsequent example (Figures 37a and b) is from a patient whose pulmonary veins have a relatively less divergent insertion into the left atrium and a smaller common confluence. In such cases, the PV angiograms and ICE would have a closer correlation.

With our technique the circular catheter is "roving" while looking for potentials around the antrum, rather than sitting at a fixed spot (Figure 6.38). The diameter of the circular mapping catheter used does not bear any relation to the size of the pulmonary vein. Owing to the relatively asymmetric and oblique orientation of the funnel-shaped portion of the left superior and inferior pulmonary veins on the ICE longitudinal view, the anterior segments appear slightly deeper into the antrum. Figures 6.39 to 6.43 are serial images of corresponding fluoroscopic and ICE images showing

the circular mapping catheter as it is used to guide the ablation catheter along the various segments of the left superior and inferior pulmonary venous antrum. We usually start the procedure along the anterior segment of the left superior pulmonary vein as shown in Figure 6.38a and b. The catheter is then navigated around the antrum of the LSPV and LIPV to achieve isolation along their superior, posterior, and inferior aspects. The corresponding fluoroscopy and ICE pictures along these aspects are shown in Figures 6.40 to 6.43. This area corresponds to the end of the tube-like portion of the pulmonary vein, as shown in Figures 6.3 and 6.5. Usually at this position energy is applied only at the roof, the carina, and the anterior segments. The anterior segments correspond to the ridge of tissue between the appendage and the left superior PV. Ablation in this area is challenging and requires significant skill and experience.

The corresponding electrograms in this position, before and after ablation are shown in Figures 6.39c and d. Figures 6.57a and 6.25b are examples of two patients where electroanatomic maps of the left atrium were obtained. The yellow dots represent the border of the pulmonary vein ostium, as defined by CARTO. The operator was then blinded to help the

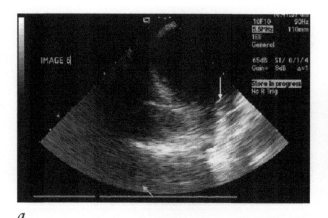

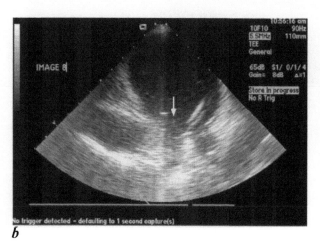

Figure 6.37 *(a,b) The circular catheter in the left superior pulmonary vein (LSPV) and the left inferior pulmonary vein (LIPV) in a patient with a short common confluence.*

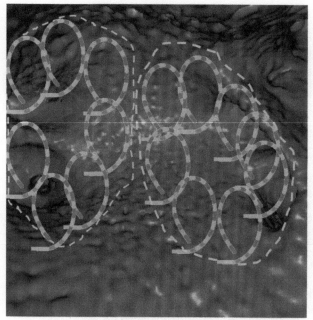

Figure 6.38 *Schematic representation of the various placements of the circular mapping catheter as it is used to help isolate the antrum of the left and the right pulmonary veins, respectively. Note that the circular lines around the posterior wall of the left atrium on the two sides often merge with each other. Therefore, in most cases, the posterior wall represents the confluence of the antrum of the four pulmonary veins.*

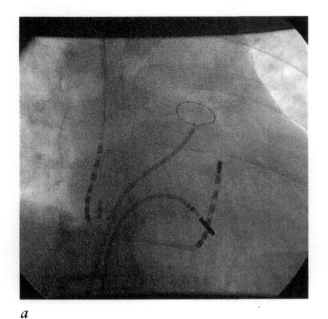

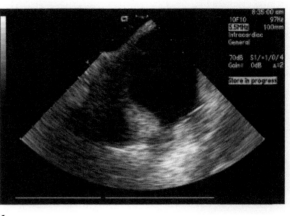

a   *b*

Figures 6.39a,b   *Simultaneous fluoroscopic and ICE pictures of the circular mapping catheter at the initial position during isolation of the antrum of the left superior pulmonary vein. The circular catheter, on the ICE, is placed at the level of the tubular portion of the pulmonary veins. The simultaneous anterior position of the catheter is appreciable on the RAO view of the fluoroscopy too. In this position, only the anterior, anterosuperior segments of the antrum, and the carina (junction with the left inferior pulmonary vein) are isolated. The antrum has to be visualized as an oblique/ellipsoid-shaped opening with the most proximal portion displaced posteriorly and the anterior segments represented by the borders of the tubular part of the vein.*

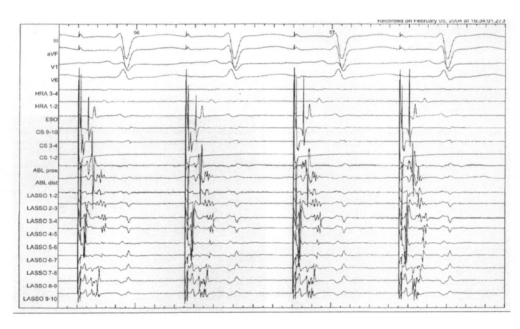

c

Figure 6.39c,d   *Continued.*

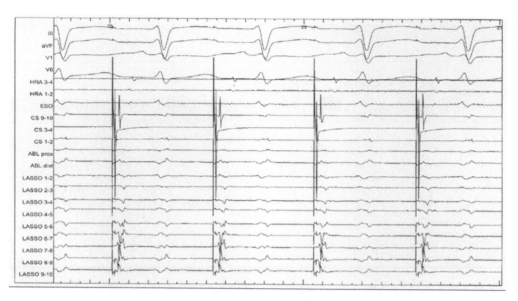

d

Figure 6.39c,d *(c) The ICE recordings from the circular mapping catheter along the anterior segments of the left superior pulmonary vein antrum from the position corresponding to Figures 6.39a and b. Note the separation of the high-frequency pulmonary vein potentials during pacing from the distal coronary sinus. (d) After ablation, abolition of all pulmonary vein potentials, which is our endpoint for the isolation of the respective segment, is shown. The high-amplitude signals from the left atrial appendage are seen to persist even after the ablation and are important to differentiate from the pulmonary vein potentials along the anterior segment.*

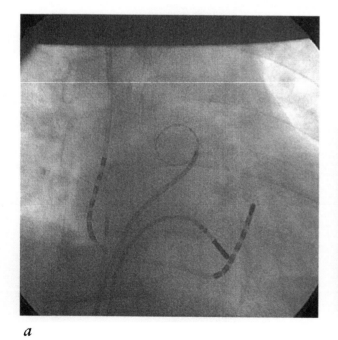

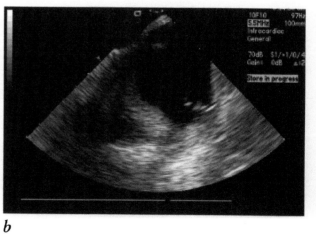

a   b

Figures 6.40a,b *The catheter has now been moved more posteriorly and this can be easily appreciated on the fluoroscopic view. The ICE picture shows that the catheter is now placed more proximally at the level of the funnel-shaped portion of the pulmonary vein.*

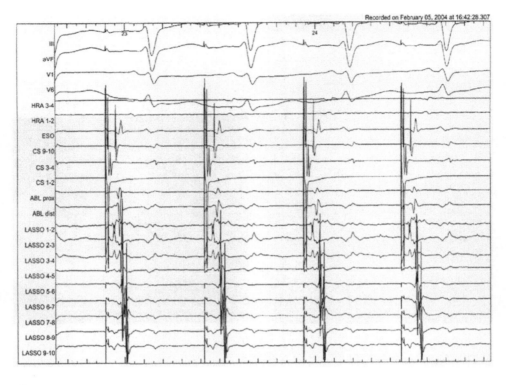

c

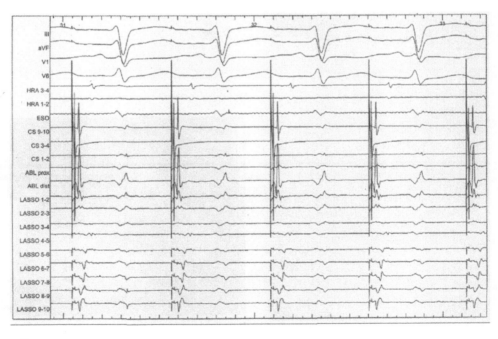

d

Figure 6.40c,d   *(c) The ICE recordings from the more posterior segments of the left superior pulmonary vein (LSPV) correspond to the position of the circular mapping catheter in Figures 6.40a and 6.40b. The potentials along the posterior wall are of a higher amplitude and frequency when compared to those along the anterior segments of the vein. Pacing from the distal coronary sinus (CS) is useful in separating them from the low-frequency, low-amplitude atrial signals which are seen to persist after the ablation (d).*

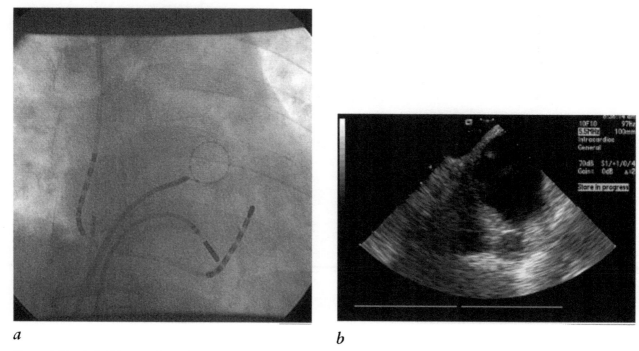

a   *b*

Figure 6.41   *(a,b) The circular catheter has been moved in the left inferior pulmonary vein (LIPV) at the level of the tubular portion. This position is important to isolate the anterior portions of the antrum, including the carina (roof of the tubular portion of the LIPV), anterior segments, and the inferior margin of the tubular portion of the vein.*

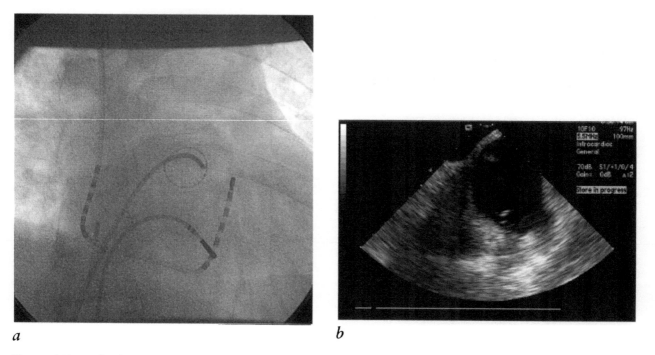

a   *b*

Figures 6.42   *(a,b) Placement of the circular catheter in the more posterior and inferior aspect of the antrum of the left inferior pulmonary vein.*

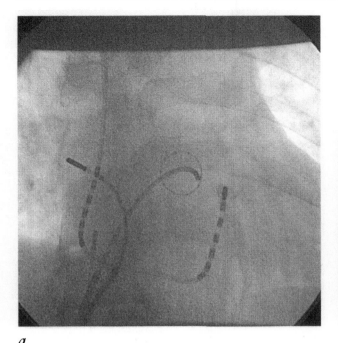

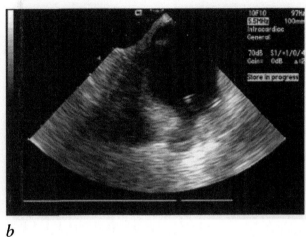

a   *b*

Figures 6.43 *(a,b) This set of pictures shows a slightly superior and posterior shift of the circular mapping catheter in comparison to the previous image. The catheter is now moved to cover the more posterior edges of the antrum. Once the various segments of the LSPV and LIPV antrum have been isolated, the final line of block that is achieved corresponds to a wide area around these veins, as shown in Figure 6.44.*

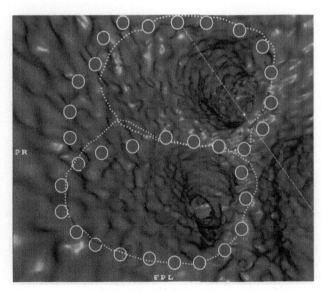

Figure 6.44 *A pictographic representation of the intended movements of the circular mapping catheter as it is navigated to guide the ablation along the antrum of the left superior and left inferior pulmonary veins in Figures 6.40–6.43. The dashed blue lines represent the various positions of the circular catheter and the red dots represent the ablation points in each of these positions. The dotted yellow line corresponds to the final ablation line, which disconnects the pulmonary vein antrum from the left atrium. After isolation of the left PV antra, the catheters are moved towards the RSPV and RIPV antrum. Figures 6.45–6.51 show corresponding fluoroscopic and ICE images as the catheters are moved along the various segments of the right PV antra.*

electroanatomic map, and ablation was performed using ICE. The ablation points (labeled as red) were tagged during the procedure on a separate map and then superimposed on the previous map. Ablation guided by ICE appears more proximal. In our experience, isolation of the pulmonary vein antrum is essential for complete and effective isolation of most of the triggers of atrial fibrillation.

CATHETER CONTACT AND TITRATION OF ENERGY DELIVERY

In addition to positioning the mapping catheter in the left atrium, ICE can be helpful in monitoring the catheter–tissue interface during energy delivery. Poor contact between the catheter and the tissues reduces resistive heating through the desired site and increases convective heat loss into the circulating blood. This could result in diminished heat delivery, inefficient lesion formation, and increases the risk of coagulum formation.

The contact between the catheter–tissue interface is traditionally monitored by looking for catheter stability on fluoroscopy and the quality of electrical recording. ICE can be used to evaluate catheter movement during lesion delivery without the need for intermittent fluoroscopy. Kalman et al[8] have reported that ICE can be used to improve the percentage

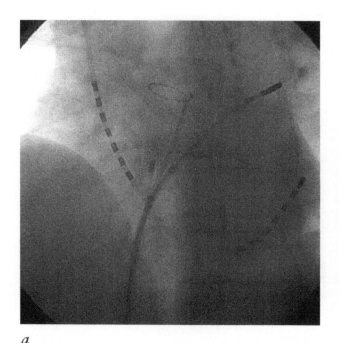

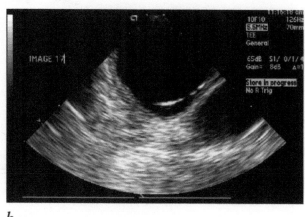

Figure 6.45(a,b)

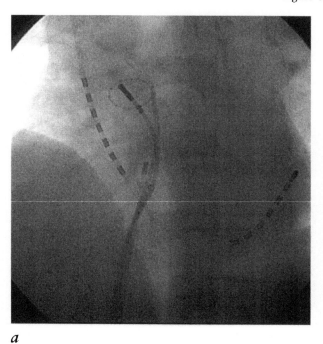

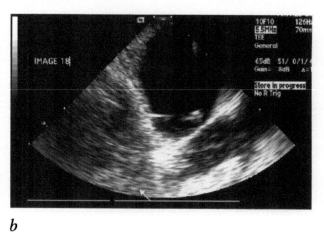

Figure 6.46(a,b)

of lesions with good contact during RF energy delivery. This can increase the lesion size and procedural success.

ICE is also useful as a monitoring tool while titrating energy delivery during RF applications. Conventionally, temperature, power, and impedance are among the various measures that are monitored during RF energy delivery. Application of RF energy

is discontinued either when adequate power is delivered at the desired temperature for a preset time or if there is any impedance rise signifying char formation. In our initial experience using ICE, we noted that impedance rise during RF energy delivery was preceded by a dense shower of microbubbles. Therefore, we have considered microbubbles to be a manifestation of tissue overheating and have devised

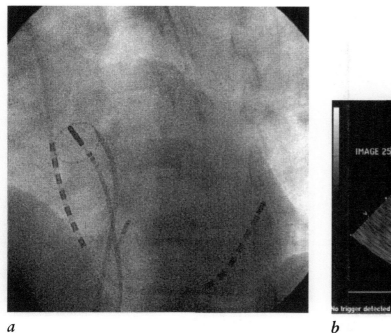

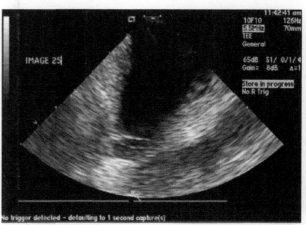

a   b

Figure 6.47(a,b)

Figures 6.45–6.48 *Simultaneous fluoroscopic and ICE pictures (a and b, respectively) of the circular mapping catheter, as it is navigated through different regions of the right superior pulmonary vein antrum. All fluoroscopic views are in shallow left anterior oblique view (LAO). In Figures 6.45a and 6.45b, the catheter is placed along the roof and is then moved towards the inferior aspect of the vein, which is in relation to the carina (Figure 6.46a,b), i.e. the junction between the superior and the inferior veins.*

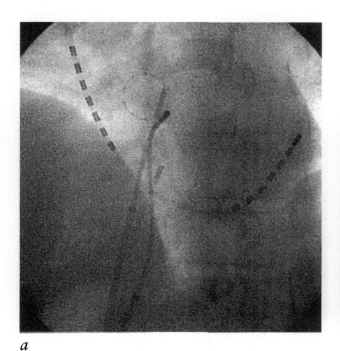

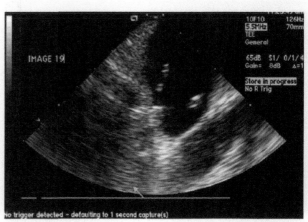

a   b

Figure 6.48(a,b) *In Figures 6.47a,b and 6.48a,b the circular catheter is moved along the septum and the posterior wall, respectively. Note how the catheter is deeply seated when placed along the septal segments (anterior) in Figure 6.47b.*

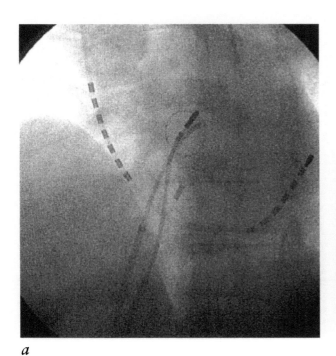

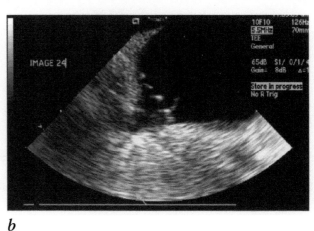

a   *b*

Figure 6.49(a,b) *After the various segments on the right sided veins have been isolated, the final area of isolation achieved is shown in Figure 6.52. The availability of image integration has made it easier to understand the anatomy in a 3D view. Figures 6.53 and 6.54 are examples of extremely high septal and anterior position at which ablation is often required to isolate the RSPV. The electrograms confirm the presence of PV potentials in this area. The subsequent example shows a 3D view of the lesions along the interior aspect of the left and right PV antra.*

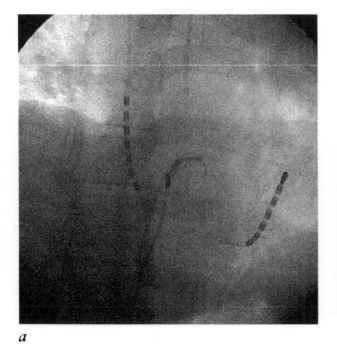

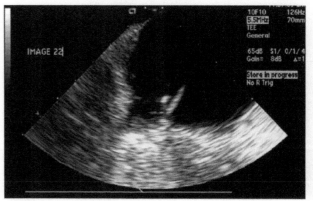

a   *b*

Figure 6.50(a,b)

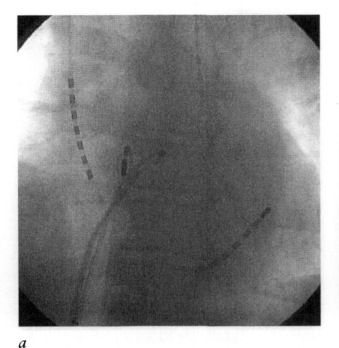

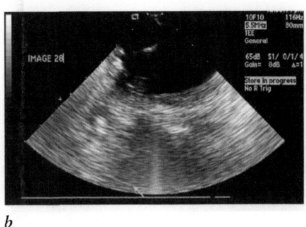

a   *b*

Figure 6.51(a,b)

Figure 6.49–6.51 *The different positions of the circular mapping catheter around the right inferior pulmonary vein antrum. All fluoroscopic views are in a shallow left anterior oblique view (LAO). Figure 6.49a,b shows the catheter inside the ostium of this relatively short and tubular vein, which is located slightly inferior and posterior to the right superior pulmonary vein (RSPV). Note that despite significant movement of the catheter on fluoroscopy, towards the posterior and the septal aspects in Figures 6.50a,b and 6.51a,b, respectively, the ICE shows that the circular catheter remains around the ostium of the RIPV. This again exemplifies the importance of "navigating" the circular catheter around the pulmonary vein antrum, to achieve complete isolation of this region whereby both ICE and fluoroscopy are complementary and important.*

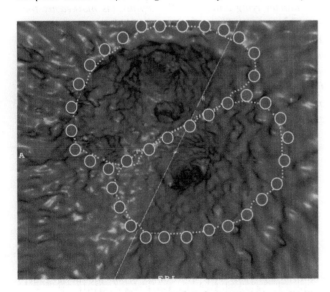

Figure 6.52 *A three-dimensional endoscopic reconstruction of the right pulmonary veins. The seven positions of the circular mapping catheter (as depicted for the patient in Figures 6.45–6.51) are shown in dashed blue lines. The red dots represent the intended ablation spots in relation to the border of the mapping catheter while targeting the pulmonary vein potentials recorded from its surface. The dotted yellow lines represent the final ablation lines along which isolation of the right pulmonary vein antra is achieved.*

an RF energy delivery protocol during which power is titrated down or RF application is discontinued as soon as microbubbles are seen on ICE. By guiding our ablation using microbubble formation to titrate power output, we have seen improved success rates and reduced risk of complications.[4]

Radiofrequency energy is delivered starting at 25–30 W, keeping a target temperature of 55°C. The power is then titrated upwards in a gradual step-up fashion in increments of 5 W until scattered uniform bubbles are seen (Figure 6.60), and is then kept constant at about 5 W below this level. If a brisk shower of microbubbles is observed (Figures 6.61 and 6.62), energy delivery is terminated instantly. With the use of transcranial Doppler, we have also been able to demonstrate a relation between the risk of symptomatic and asymptomatic thrombo-embolic episodes and the formation/frequency of microbubbles (Figure 6.63). Recently, we have also noted that there may be a relation between the incidence of microbubble formation and temperature rise in the esophagus. Hence, we believe that monitoring for microbubbles and titrating energy delivery with our protocol may be helpful in reducing the risk of left atrial–esophageal fistulas and embolic complications.

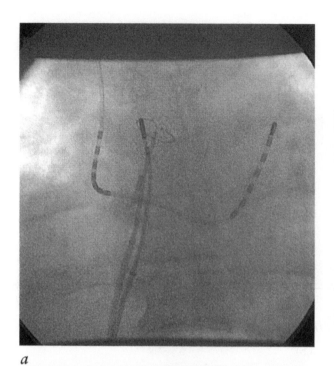

a

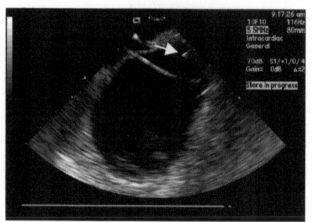

b

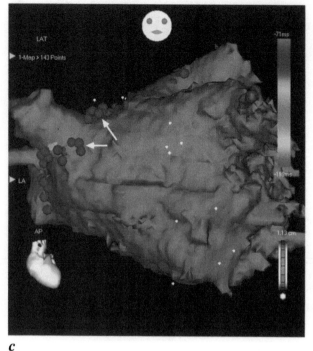

c

Figures 6.53   *Examples showing very anterior/septal lesions which are required to isolate the right pulmonary veins antrum. (a) The picture in the left anterior oblique (LAO) fluoroscopic view in this patient shows the circular mapping catheter placed very anterior in relation to the right superior pulmonary vein. (b) ICE confirms the position and shows the catheter lying almost on the septum (as marked by the white arrow). (c) The view from CARTO merge shows the ablation lesions (marked by black arrows) that were placed very anterior, almost on the posterosuperior aspect of the interatrial septum. This site showed well-defined high-frequency pulmonary vein potentials, and their isolation as anterior, as the ICE and CARTO merge pictures show, is essential to successfully isolate the right PV antrum.*

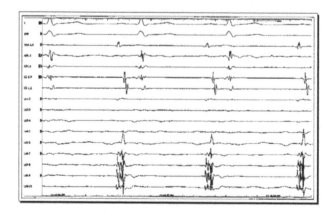

Figure 6.54   *The ICE recordings from the above site, confirming the presence of high-frequency pulmonary vein potentials along the electrodes LS7-10 on the circular mapping catheter. Ablation along these electrodes resulted in abolition of these high-frequency potentials and isolation of this segment of the right superior pulmonary vein antrum.*

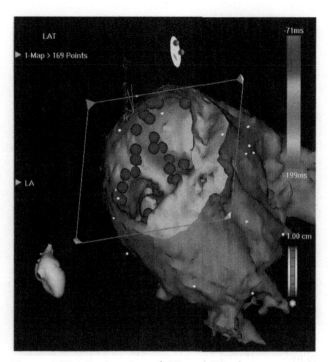

Figure 6.55 *Registration of CT and 3D electro-anatomic mapping in a right lateral–caudal view. The left-sided pulmonary veins are visible from the inside. The red dots represent the ablation lesions that have been delivered to isolate the left pulmonary venous antrum.*

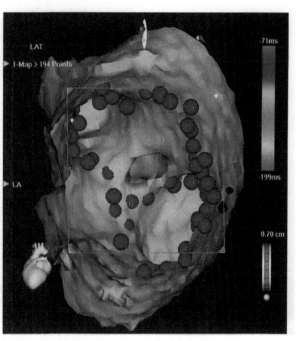

Figure 6.56 *An endoscopic view of the right superior and inferior pulmonary veins. The 3D CT image of the left atrium is registered on a mapping system for navigation and ablation. Multiple lesions over a wide area were delivered to isolate the pulmonary venous antrum of both veins. Note that the right middle lobe vein is incorporated within the lesions of the right superior pulmonary vein antrum.*

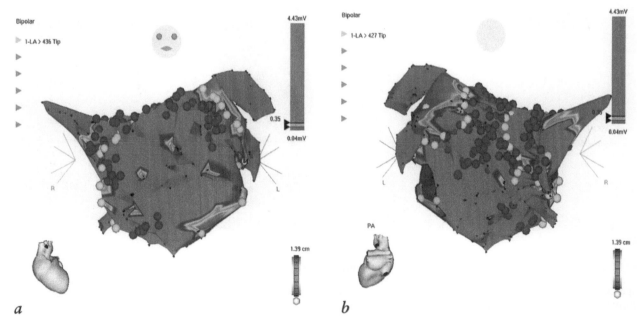

a   *b*

Figure 6.57 *(a, b) A comparison in the definition of the ostia of the pulmonary veins by 3D electro-anatomic mapping versus ICE. The anterior and posterior views show the ostial points as defined by CARTO (yellow tags) and by ICE (red ablation tags). The ICE-guided ablation is far more proximal than the points defined by electro-anatomic mapping alone, especially posteriorly. The posterior view again exemplifies how the two lesion sets around the right and the left pulmonary venous antrum usually merge with each other. ICE can sometimes be very useful in confirming the ostial locations in patients with an unusual anatomy. Some of these situations were discussed earlier, but another example, where fluoroscopic positions could be deceptive, is shown in Figures 6.58 and 6.59.*

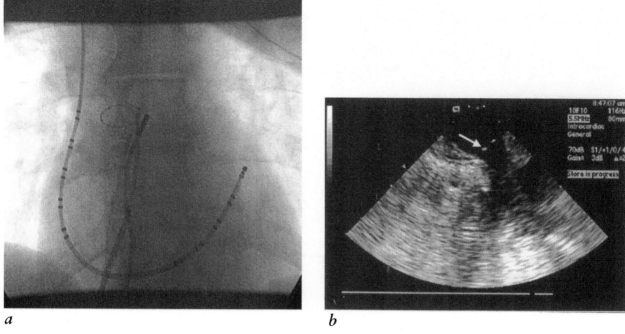

Figure 6.58(a,b)

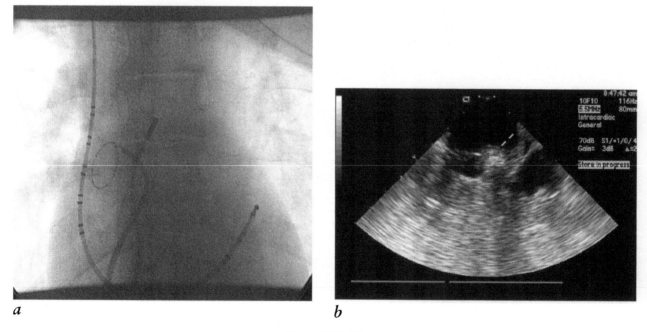

Figure 6.59(a,b)

Figures 6.58 and 6.59   *Examples from a patient who had an unusual vertical take-off of the right superior pulmonary vein (RSPV) and, subsequently, a high-take off of the right inferior pulmonary vein (RIPV). Figure 6.58a shows the fluoroscopic image of the circular catheter at the ostium of the tubular portion of the RSPV. In most situations, this would appear to be placed along the roof of the left atrium in relation to the vein. However, the ICE image in Figure 6.58b confirms that the catheter is at the ostium of the RSPV (as marked by the white arrow). The long axis of the RSPV can be appreciated in relation to the right pulmonary artery, which in turn is seen in the far-field view of the picture. Figure 6.59a shows the left anterior oblique (LAO) fluoroscopic view of the catheter at the ostium of the RIPV. This looks much higher than usual, and in fact, corresponds to the usual position of the RSPV. The ICE image in Figure 6.59b confirms that the catheter is at the ostium of the RIPV, as shown by the red arrow. The ostium of the RSPV is shown by the yellow dashed line on the right of the scan.*

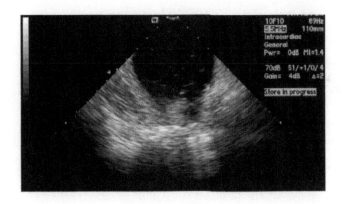

Figure 6.60 *The long-axis view of the left superior and left inferior pulmonary veins. The circular mapping catheter, as shown by the yellow arrow, is positioned at the ostium of the left superior pulmonary vein. There are scattered microbubbles visualized as small white particles within the left atrial cavity.*

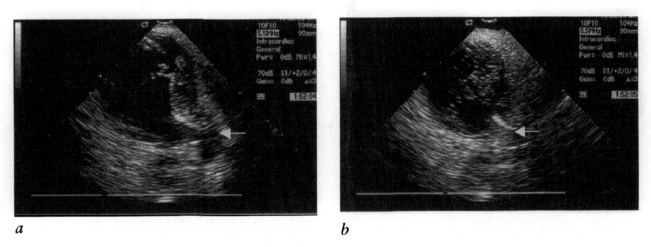

a   *b*

Figure 6.61 *(a,b) A brisk shower of microbubbles during delivery of radiofrequency (RF) energy. The yellow arrows depict the catheter tip–tissue interface. The microbubbles originate from the tip of the catheter and then spread out into the left atrial cavity.*

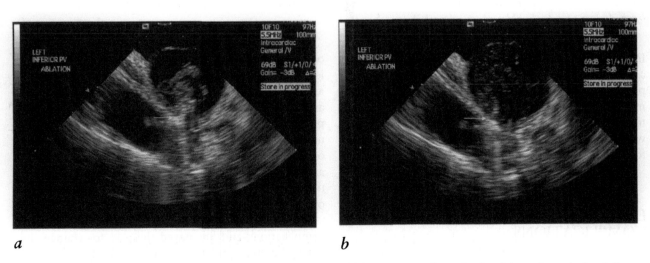

a   *b*

Figure 6.62 *(a,b) Another example of a dense shower of microbubbles emanating from the tip of the catheter during delivery of radiofrequency (RF) energy. In such situations, RF energy delivery is immediately terminated. The yellow arrows show the tip of the ablation catheter.*

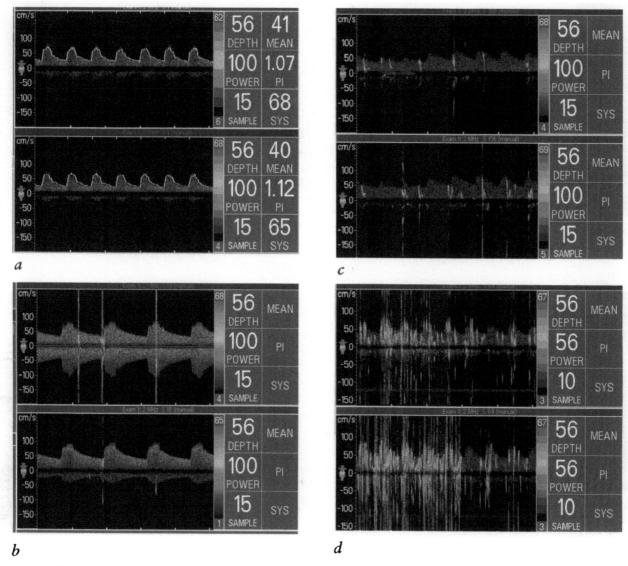

Figures 6.63 *Examples of the transcranial Doppler flow recordings during ablation. (a) At baseline, the normal undisturbed uniphasic flow in the right and left middle cerebral artery. (b) A recording during a few scattered microbubbles on ICE, showing occasional turbulence that reflects microembolic signals (MES). (c) It is easy to appreciate the increasing turbulence during a modest rise in the microbubbles. (d) Increased density of MES is recorded on the transcranial Doppler during a brisk shower of microbubbles observed on ICE.*

Interestingly, the formation of microbubbles has a very variable pattern and is not governed by specific power settings or temperature readings. In animal models, microbubble formation has been confirmed to be associated with tissue overheating. Clinically, we have also seen a relationship between microbubble formation and certain complications.

EARLY DETECTION OF COMPLICATIONS

Transthoracic echocardiography has limitations in terms of resolution and depth of information. The use of transesophageal echocardiography carries significant discomfort and the risk of bleeding and aspiration. ICE overcomes some of these limitations and the phased-array probes can be safely manipulated within the right atrium itself, without the need to cross the interatrial septum. Advancement of the ICE probe could result in vascular injury and/or perforation. We have not seen these complications, but the need for caution cannot be overemphasized.

ICE imaging has been important in detecting complications and has paved the way for changes in anticoagulation and power titration protocols. Some of the examples of how ICE has been helpful in the early detection and management of complications are shown in Figures 6.64–6.69.

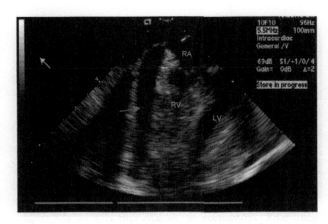

Figure 6.64 *This figure highlights a four-chamber view, showing the right ventricle (RV), the right atrium (RA), and a part of the left ventricle (LV) and left atrium. The red arrow depicts an echo-free space anterior to the RV, which suggests the presence of pericardial effusion noted during the procedure. Evidence of RV/RA diastolic collapse suggestive of cardiac tamponade was noted before any hemodynamic instability and the patient underwent successful pericardiocentesis. The green arrow shows a small fluid collection posterior to the LV.*

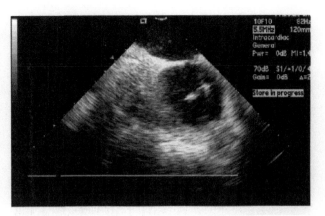

Figure 6.65 *A mobile thrombus on the sheath in the left atrium (as marked by the red arrow). These usually form on the transseptal sheath, but rarely on the mapping and ablation catheter. They are most often noted when the activated coagulation time (ACT) is below 350 s and within a few minutes after entering the left atrium. Based on this observation, confirmed by other groups, we administer intravenous heparin before the transseptal puncture. The sheaths are also continuously flushed with heparinized saline. An intravenous infusion of heparin is used to maintain the ACT around 400 s.*

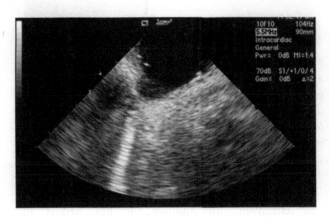

Figure 6.66 *Example of a complication observed after episodes of dense microbubbles were ignored. In this patient, one can visualize endothelial disruption and charry thrombus formation at the ostium of the right inferior pulmonary vein where radiofrequency energy was delivered.*

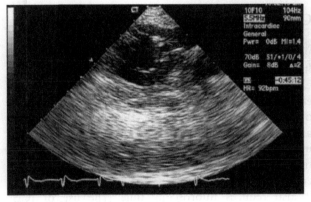

a

Figure 6.67a *Echo-dense material on the body of the circular mapping catheter. It is uncommon for thrombi to form on these catheters with adequate anticoagulation, as it is constantly in motion in the left atrium. Most often, this echo-dense material is char formation, which develops with tissue overheating and is often associated with frequent episodes of microbubble formation. This material is adherent to the catheter. Hence, the catheter can usually be pulled back carefully in the sheath and the material can be withdrawn with the syringe. The catheter is then cleaned and the sheaths cleared before reintroducing the catheters in the left atrium.*

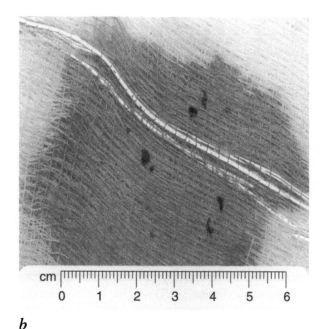

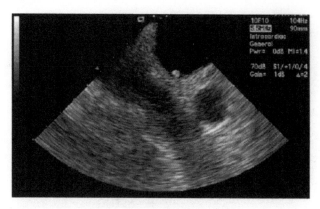

Figure 6.68 *Formation of an adherent clot on the atrial endocardium in a patient undergoing isolation of the right pulmonary vein antrum. This occurred immediately after a dense shower of microbubbles.*

b

Figure 6.67b *Debris that was aspirated from the sheath in the patient in Figure 6.67a, who had recurrent impedance rise, shower of microbubbles, and formation of echo-dense material on the mapping catheter. The incidence of this has dramatically reduced since we have started using ICE to monitor for microbubble formation during energy delivery.*

CONCLUSION

It is evident that ICE plays an important role during catheter ablation for atrial fibrillation. It is a safe and effective modality which provides real-time imaging of the complex anatomy of the pulmonary veins and the left atrium. It helps in quickly identifying anatomic variations and provides online visualization for placement of the mapping and ablation catheters and monitoring their position. Hence, it also reduces fluoroscopy time. The use of ICE has been critical in teaching us about procedural complications so that they can be managed timely

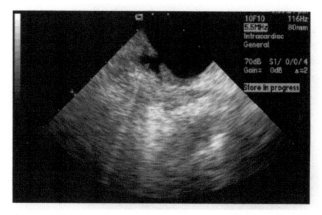

Figure 6.69 *Another unusual complication, which was seen after a brisk shower of microbubbles. A crater formed in the wall of the left atrium, adjacent to the ostium of the right inferior pulmonary vein. The above complications can be minimized by titrating energy while monitoring for microbubble formation.*

and effectively. In addition, it has helped in developing safer anticoagulation and energy delivery protocols.

REFERENCES

1. Haissaguerre M, Jais P, Shah DC, et al. Spontaneous initiation of atrial fibrillation by ectopic beats originating in the pulmonary veins. N Engl J Med 1998; 339: 659–66.
2. Perez-Lugones A, McMahon JT, Ratliff NB, et al. Evidence of specialized conduction cells in human pulmonary veins of patients with atrial fibrillation. J Cardiovasc Electrophysiol 2003; 14: 803–9.
3. Jalife J, Berenfeld O, Mansour M. Mother rotors and fibrillatory conduction: a mechanism of atrial fibrillation. Cardiovasc Res 2002; 54: 204–16.
4. Marrouche NF, Martin DO, Wazni O, et al. Phased-array intracardiac echocardiography monitoring during pulmonary vein isolation in patients with atrial fibrillation: impact on outcome and complications. Circulation 2003; 107: 2710–16.

5. Verma A, Marrouche NF, Yamada H, et al. Usefulness of intracardiac Doppler assessment of left atrial function immediately post-pulmonary vein antrum isolation to predict short-term recurrence of atrial fibrillation. Am J Cardiol 2004; 94: 951.

6. Saad EB, Cole CR, Marrouche NF, et al. Use of intracardiac echocardiography for prediction of chronic pulmonary vein stenosis after ablation of atrial fibrillation. J Cardiovasc Electrophysiol 2002; 13(10): 986–9.

7. Ren JF, Marchlinski FE, Callans DJ, Zado ES. Intracardiac Doppler echocardiographic quantification of pulmonary vein flow velocity: an effective technique for monitoring pulmonary vein ostia narrowing during focal atrial fibrillation ablation. J Cardiovasc Electrophysiol 2002; 13: 1076–81.

8. Kalman JM, Fitzpatrick AP, Olgin JE, et al. Biophysical characteristics of radiofrequency lesion formation in vivo: dynamics of catheter tip–tissue contact evaluated by intracardiac echocardiography. Am Heart J 1997; 133: 8–18.

Chapter 7 Transcatheter occlusion of left atrial appendage for stroke prevention in atrial fibrillation – potential role for intracardiac echocardiography

Hsuan-Hung Chuang, Dhanunjaya Lakkireddy, Jennifer Cummings, and E Murat Tuzcu

INTRODUCTION

Atrial fibrillation (AF), a leading cause of hospitalization among the elderly, is the most common arrhythmia encountered by clinicians, with an estimated prevalence of 0.4% in the general population. AF is associated with a high risk for thromboembolic stroke. In patients with non-rheumatic AF, the incidence of embolic stroke is 2- to 7-fold higher, with a mortality rate that is twice that of people in normal sinus rhythm. About 30% of all patients with ischemic stroke or transient ischemic attack are found to have a potential cardiac source of embolism.[1] The left atrial appendage (LAA) is the source of the vast majority of these thromboemboli.[2]

Oral anticoagulation (OAC) significantly reduces the rate of stroke or embolism in patients with AF.[3] Although OAC has been shown to be safe and effective, it is often difficult to achieve a well-controlled therapeutic range of anticoagulation over long periods of time.[4] Moreover, more than 50% of the AF population are aged 75 years old or older, with 20% or more having a contraindication to OAC.[5] In practice, only about one-third of the eligible patients actually receive OAC therapy continuously and effectively as per recommendation.[5–7]

There has been a shift towards catheter-based interventional techniques following the success of surgical Maze procedures, which cure AF in >90% of patients and virtually eliminate the risk of stroke.[8] Radiofrequency ablation and pulmonary vein isolation has been reported a success in 70–80% of patients.[9] However, from the standpoint of stroke prevention, it is unrealistic to expect to cure all or most AF patients with percutaneous or surgical treatments. Surgical obliteration of the LAA has proven its effectiveness in eliminating the predilection of this site for thrombus formation.[2,10,11] It may be performed as an additional procedure during cardiac valve or coronary bypass surgery,[12] as part of the Maze procedure,[13] or as an isolated procedure via thoracoscopy.[10,14] Although the complete obliteration of the LAA is the surgical goal, residual communication between the left atrium (LA) cavity and the LAA has been reported in as many as 36% of patients after mitral valve surgery.[15] Thrombi within an incompletely ligated LAA may occur and embolize.[16] An alternative modality of treatment – percutaneous mechanical occlusion of the LAA – has emerged in recent years,[17–19] and mid-term results from limited animal and human studies have been encouraging.

Transesophageal echocardiography (TEE) has been an integral part in the evaluation of patients with suspected cardioembolic cerebrovascular events, and in providing guidance during interventional procedures. Intracardiac echocardiography (ICE), a new invasive imaging modality, shows great potential in enhancing periprocedural imaging, including percutaneous occlusion of the LAA in the secondary prevention of cardioembolic stroke.

ANATOMY AND FUNCTION OF THE LEFT ATRIAL APPENDAGE

The LAA, the embryologic remnant of the left atrium, develops during the third week of gestation. The main LA cavity develops later and is formed from the outgrowth of the pulmonary veins. The LAA is a muscular extension that projects anterolaterally between the left upper pulmonary vein and the left ventricle.[20,21] There is a high degree of variability in the morphology of the LAA (Figure 7.1). The diameter of the orifice of the LAA is about 10–40 mm. The LAA is multilobulated in 80% of human hearts, formed by three lobules in 23% and by four lobules in 3% of cases.[20] The lobules can lie in an anatomic plane different from the main tubular body. Al-Saady et al[22] found that in 70% of the cases, the main axis of LAA is markedly bent or spiral, accounting for the differences in shape and size when viewed through 2D echocardiography. Patients with AF macroscopically had significantly larger LAA volumes, larger luminal surfaces, and less pectinate muscle compared with those with sinus rhythm.[21,23] Microscopically, there were more endocardial thickening with fibrous and elastic tissue, fibrosis, myocyte hypertrophy, myocyte dystrophy with myolysis, and apoptosis. These features of LAA remodeling in AF serve as the substrate for electrical remodeling, whereby the atrial effective refractory period shortens and impairs its rate adaptive response.[24]

The LAA function depends on complex factors such as age, heart rate, rhythm, and loading conditions. It plays an important role in the maintenance and regulation of the cardiac function, in hypertension, AF, valvular heart disease, and heart failure. LAA dysfunction, as a risk factor in thrombus formation and stroke in patients with AF/atrial flutter and mitral valve

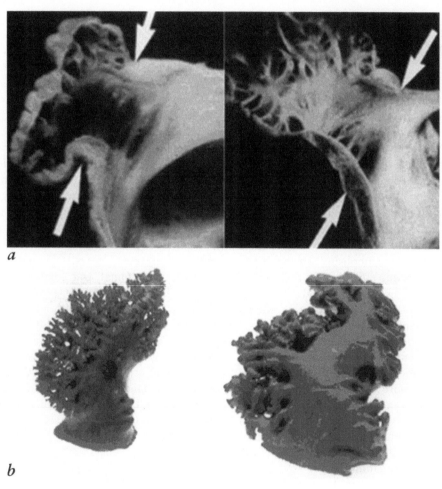

Figure 7.1 *(a) Pathologic specimens of the left atrial appendage (LAA). Bilobed LAA on the left and multilobed LAA on the right. (b) Postmortem LAA casts. The cast on the left side is from a 52-year-old man who had antemortem sinus rhythm. The cast volume is 5.880 cm³. The cast has more than five branches and 20–40 twigs, and is densely covered with fine structures. The cast on the right side is from a 76-year-old woman who had antemortem atrial fibrillation. The cast volume is 18.670 cm³. The cast has more than five branches, >40 twigs, and no fine structures. (Reproduced with permission from Agmon et al. Echocardiographic assessment of the left atrial appendage. J Am Coll Cardiol 1999; 34: 1867–77; and Stollberger et al. Elimination of the left atrial appendage to prevent stroke or embolism? Anatomic, physiologic, and pathophysiologic considerations. Chest 2003; 124: 2356–62.)*

disease, is well documented.[25,26] LAA dysfunction is, likewise, found in patients with reduced ventricular function and elevated LA pressures. In patients with sinus rhythm, reduction of LAA function is uncommon (7%).[27] Decreased contractile function of the LAA can lead to blood stasis and formation of thrombi.[28,29] In clinical practice, LAA function is determined primarily based on the flow velocities and area change.

Although the mechanical occlusion of the LAA appears a reasonable alternative to OAC in the treatment of AF, especially in patients with contraindications to OAC therapy, further studies will be needed to assess the long-term effect as well as the neurohormonal and hemodynamic consequences. Tabata et al[30] showed that in humans undergoing cardiac surgery for coronary heart disease or mitral regurgitation, the clamping of the LAA led to an increase in diastolic transmitral and pulmonary flow velocities, and to an increase in LA mean pressure and size. In studies with patients who had undergone the Maze procedure and bilateral atrial appendectomy had been performed, attenuation of natriuretic peptide secretion and water retention were found in the early postoperative phase.[31,32]

MECHANICAL OCCLUSION OF THE LEFT ATRIAL APPENDAGE

Most of the experience has been with the PLAATO (percutaneous left atrial appendage transcatheter occlusion) system (Appriva Medical, Inc., Sunnyvale, CA). The newer device that is currently used in clinical trials is the Watchman device, as shown in Figure 7.2. Animal studies demonstrated the ability of the device to mechanically occlude the LAA. The PLAATO device consists of a self-expanding balloon-shaped nitinol cage with an expanded polytetrafluoroethylene (ePTFE) membrane. The membrane covers the atrial surface of the device, whereas the opposite surface is not covered, thereby allowing for thrombosis of the lumen of the device.

The device is introduced via a femoral venous sheath and advanced into the LAA following transseptal puncture of the interatrial septum (IAS). The transseptal puncture is mostly performed under fluoroscopic guidance using established radiographic landmarks that allow a correct location of the IAS in the majority of cases. Continuous hemodynamic pressure monitoring adds to the safety of the procedure. The landmarks might be misleading when there is distortion of the atrial or septal anatomy in conditions such as LA dilation and atrial septum aneurysm, and thereby increase the risk of complications such as atrial free wall puncture. Transesophageal echocardiography or intracardiac echocardiography may be helpful in such

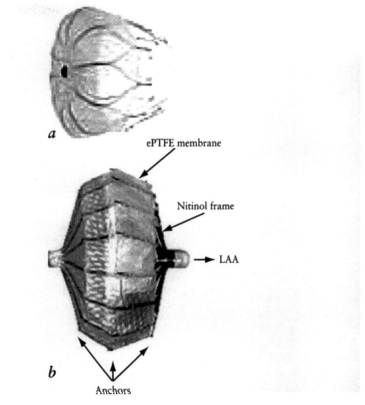

Figure 7.2 *Two different left atrial appendage occluder devices: (a) the Watchman device (reproduced with the permission of Hein R et al. Patent foramen ovale and left atrial appendage: new devices and methods or closure. Pediatr Cardiology. 2005 May–Jun; 26(3): 234–40); and (b) the PLAATO device (reproduced with the permission of Nakai T et al. Percutaneous Left Atrial Appendage Occlusion (PLAATO) for Preventing Cardioembolism. Circulation 2002; 105: 2217). LAA = left atrial appendage; ePTFE = expanded polytetrafluoroethylene.*

patients. Patients are given heparin after the transseptal puncture in order to keep the activated clotting time (ACT) >250 s. Prior to delivery of the device, the morphology of the LAA can be assessed by contrast injection on fluoroscopy – right anterior oblique (RAO) and anteroposterior (AP) views – and on echocardiography, and the LAA dimensions (diameter and length) measured at the end of atrial diastole.[18] The device size selected is usually 20–40% larger than the measured diameter of the LAA orifice. The delivery catheter, which contains the device, is then placed into the LAA, and then withdrawn, revealing the device, which is allowed to expand from its collapsed state to fill the appendage. The two subsequent steps will determine if the device can be released. First, contrast is injected distally into the lumen of the device, and proximally into the LA, to assess for position, effective occlusion, and any retrograde leak from the LAA (Figures 7.3–7.6). The stability of the device can be

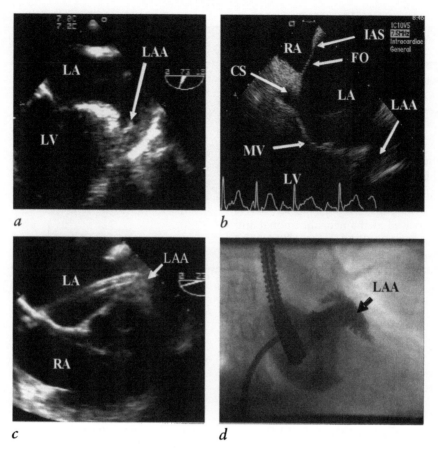

Figure 7.3 *Visualization of LAA. (a) Transesophageal view demonstrating LAA. (b) Equivalent views on intracardiac echocardiography. Injection of contrast through the transseptal sheath for identification and measurement of LAA by echocardiography (c) and fluoroscopy (d). LAA = left atrial appendage; LA = left atrium; LV = left ventricle; RA = right atrium; IAS = interatrial septum; FO = foramen ovale; CS = coronary sinus; MV = mitral valve.*

confirmed by gently tugging before it is fully released. Until the final release, the device is completely retrievable. Following the withdrawal of the introducer sheath, a repeat echocardiographic scan is performed to assess the final position of the device, the residual atrial septal defect, the pulmonary venous flow and to screen for any complications. The imaging was mainly done by using TEE (Figure 7.6), but ICE can also provide excellent pictures of the LAA (Figure 7.7). Following the procedure, patients are placed on acetylsalicylic acid (aspirin) 300 mg daily, indefinitely, and clopidogrel 75 mg daily for 6 months.

ROLE OF TRANSESOPHAGEAL AND INTRACARDIAC ECHOCARDIOGRAPHY

The LAA is optimally visualized by TEE including 2D, 3D, and Doppler techniques.[33,34] Other imaging

modalities, such as cardiac computed tomography (CT) scanning or magnetic resonance imaging (MRI), are not able to adequately visualize the LAA because of its complex morphology. As mentioned earlier, LAA varies greatly in volume and shape, and one should consider the variability when interpreting the images of LAA and planning for interventional procedures. TEE is a semi-invasive procedure and it is not entirely free of complications. The drawbacks to TEE are:

- it is uncomfortable to the patient,
- it may require general anesthesia, especially if the procedural time is long,
- it requires an additional expert operator.

ICE constitutes a new ultrasonographic modality for examination of the cardiovascular system, and has been proposed as an alternative method to guide percutaneous device closure. It was originally used to guide transseptal catheterization and radiofrequency ablation, as it allows a direct visualization of the IAS and its relation with nearby structures, and of the

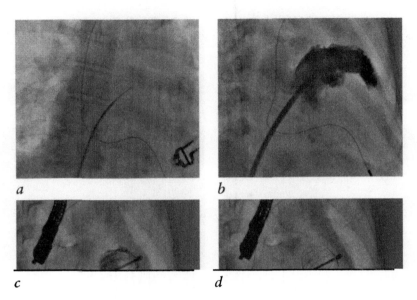

Figure 7.4 *Fluoroscopic sequence 1: (a) transseptal puncture; (b) left atrial appendage angiogram outlines the appendage and allows measurement of ostial diameter; (c) device deployed and followed by contrast injection via lumen through the implant, showing the retention of contrast behind the sealing surface; (d) stability test before release of device.*

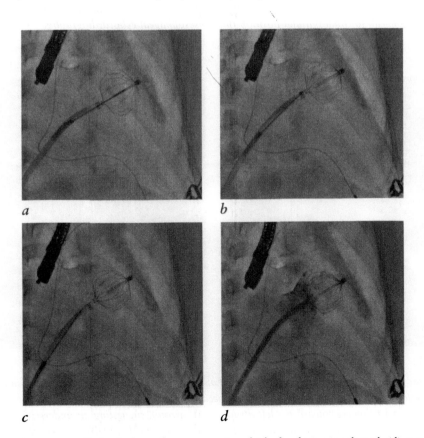

Figure 7.5 *Fluoroscopic sequence 2: (a–c) show the sequence in which the device is released; (d) contrast injection in left atrium, following device release, to confirm complete seal.*

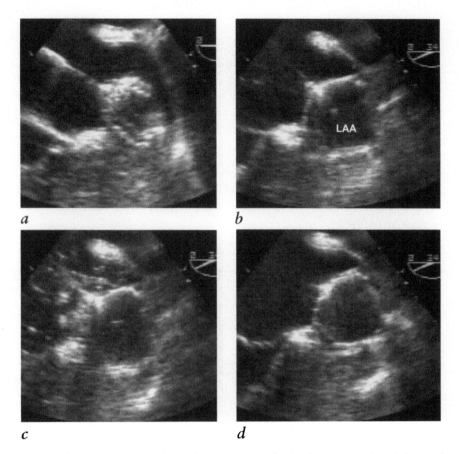

Figure 7.6 *Echocardiographic sequence: (a) device being expanded; (b) device seated in left atrial appendage (LAA); (c) contrast confirmed tight seal; (d) final optimal position on transesophageal echocardiography.*

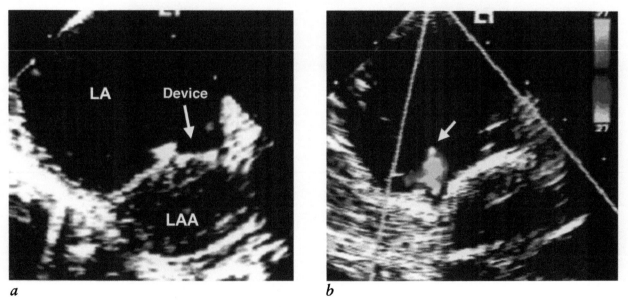

Figure 7.7 *Intracardiac echocardiographic images. (a) The left atrial appendage (LAA) with the device in place. The expanded polytetrafluoroethylene (ePTFE) membrane is echo-reflective because of microscopic trapped air. (b) A leak was detected by color Doppler imaging as a jet flowing toward the left atrium (LA) (arrow), suggesting an undersized implant. (Reproduced with permission from Nakai et al. Percutaneous left atrial appendage occlusion (PLAATO) for preventing cardioembolism: first experience in canine model. Circulation 2002; 105: 2217–22.)*

interaction between the interventional instruments and the anatomic structures. At present, intracardiac imaging may be performed by using a transducer with mechanical or electronic scanning, mounted at the distal end of a catheter. At our center, we employ the intracardiac phased-array transducer catheter. The main advantage of the phased-array intracardiac catheter scanning system over the mechanical circumferential scanning system lies in its ability to obtain high-resolution, detailed 2D ultrasound images on contiguous structures (left-sided chambers and pulmonary veins). Limitations of the phased-array system include a decrease in lateral resolution that worsens with an increase in depth, formation of side lobes as artifacts, and "echo drop-outs" of structures localized perpendicular to the direction of exploration. Although the phased-array system can provide only cardiac images in oblique planes with respect to the thorax, quite different from the multiplanar images acquired by TEE the catheter is capable of four way articulation, thus providing images at multiple angles.

In addition to guiding transseptal puncture, one can follow the deployment of the LAA occluder device, assess the residual shunt in the IAS and monitor for complications such as pericardial effusion and thrombus formation with the use of ICE. Potentially, the whole procedure could be guided continuously without the need for general anesthesia, unlike TEE, and fluoroscopy time could be shortened. All these factors could result in much lower stress to patients than TEE. However, TEE has advantages over ICE, as it possesses multiplanar imaging capability (which is ideal, as the principal axis of LAA is extremely bent and/or spiral in 70% of cases), and it provides high spatial resolution of the posterior cardiac chambers. Thus, although ICE provides anatomic detail of LAA and other cardiac structures that facilitates cardiac intervention procedures, TEE guidance remains the gold standard, and ICE cannot be considered a first-line diagnostic modality in percutaneous closure of LAA yet, until more supporting data is available. Moreover, one must consider the increased costs of the ICE catheter, which at present is a single-use disposable item.

CONCLUSIONS

Treatment of patients in AF with OAC therapy is a time-tested technique. The advantage of OAC, compared with interventional LAA occlusion, is that it is noninvasive, reversible, and may be monitored. Other than potential drug interactions, OAC does not have hemodynamic side-effects. Percutaneous occlusion of the LAA is now feasible and safe in patients with AF and contraindications to OAC therapy; no significant neurologic complications, development of atrial thrombi or thrombus formation on the device has been reported during follow-up, and it may provide an alternative treatment. This procedure, however, does not eliminate the need for long-term antithrombotic therapy and the associated bleeding risk. In addition, one should not forget that the pathogenesis of stroke or embolism in AF patients is multifactorial and is not determined only by the presence of an LAA thrombus. Hypercoagulability, which is reported in patients with AF, will not be treated by LAA occlusion.[35] Thrombogenesis is multifocal, and ventricular thrombi, aortic, carotid, or vertebral arterial plaques, or venous thrombi via right-to-left shunting are also possible embolic sources. More data are needed regarding efficacy and long-term safety, as well as the hemodynamic and neurohormonal consequences of LAA occlusion.

Echocardiography will continue to play an important role in this validation process and is ideally suited to determining appropriate patients, guiding insertion of the devices, and tracking potential complications. Intracardiac echocardiography has added a new dimension to cardiovascular imaging in interventional cardiology. At the present time, the technology is unable to provide a wide field of view, which would facilitate better user orientation within the heart and enhance navigation. New miniaturized transducers with enhanced tissue penetration and online, 3D reconstruction will be integrated in the future, which will facilitate procedures, reduce intervention and radiation times, and prevent complications.

REFERENCES

1. Cardiogenic brain embolism. The second report of the Cerebral Embolism Task Force. Arch Neurol 1989; 46: 727–43.
2. Blackshear JL, Odell JA. Appendage obliteration to reduce stroke in cardiac surgical patients with atrial fibrillation. Ann Thorac Surg 1996; 61: 755–9.
3. Risk factors for stroke and efficacy of antithrombotic therapy in atrial fibrillation. Analysis of pooled data from five randomized controlled trials. Arch Intern Med 1994; 154: 1449–57.
4. Gottlieb LK, Salem-Schatz S. Anticoagulation in atrial fibrillation. Does efficacy in clinical trials translate into effectiveness in practice? Arch Intern Med 1994; 154: 1945–53.

5. Stroke Prevention in Atrial Fibrillation Study. Final results. Circulation 1991; 84: 527–39.

6. Sudlow M, Thomson R, Thwaites B, et al. Prevalence of atrial fibrillation and eligibility for anticoagulants in the community. Lancet 1998; 352: 1167–71.

7. Bungard TJ, Ghali WA, Teo KK, et al. Why do patients with atrial fibrillation not receive warfarin? Arch Intern Med 2000; 160: 41–6.

8. Cox JL, Ad N, Palazzo T, et al. Current status of the Maze procedure for the treatment of atrial fibrillation. Semin Thorac Cardiovasc Surg 2000; 12: 15–19.

9. Gillinov AM, Blackstone EH, McCarthy PM. Atrial fibrillation: current surgical options and their assessment. Ann Thorac Surg 2002; 74: 2210–17.

10. Odell JA, Blackshear JL, Davies E, et al. Thoracoscopic obliteration of the left atrial appendage: potential for stroke reduction? Ann Thorac Surg 1996; 61: 565–9.

11. Blackshear JL, Johnson WD, Odell JA, et al. Thoracoscopic extracardiac obliteration of the left atrial appendage for stroke risk reduction in atrial fibrillation. J Am Coll Cardiol 2003; 42: 1249–52.

12. Crystal E, Lamy A, Connolly SJ, et al. Left Atrial Appendage Occlusion Study (LAAOS): a randomized clinical trial of left atrial appendage occlusion during routine coronary artery bypass graft surgery for long-term stroke prevention. Am Heart J 2003; 145: 174–8.

13. Cox JL, Boineau JP, Schuessler RB, et al. Modification of the maze procedure for atrial flutter and atrial fibrillation. I. Rationale and surgical results. J Thorac Cardiovasc Surg 1995; 110: 473–84.

14. Johnson WD, Ganjoo AK, Stone CD, et al. The left atrial appendage: our most lethal human attachment! Surgical implications. Eur J Cardiothorac Surg 2000; 17: 718–22.

15. Katz ES, Tsiamtsiouris T, Applebaum RM, et al. Surgical left atrial appendage ligation is frequently incomplete: a transesophageal echocardiographic study. J Am Coll Cardiol 2000; 36: 468–71.

16. Rosenzweig BP, Katz E, Kort S, et al. Thromboembolus from a ligated left atrial appendage. J Am Soc Echocardiogr 2001; 14: 396–8.

17. Nakai T, Lesh M, Ostermayer S, et al. An endovascular approach to cardioembolic stroke prevention in atrial fibrillation patients. Pacing Clin Electrophysiol 2003; 26: 1604–6.

18. Sievert H, Lesh MD, Trepels T, et al. Percutaneous left atrial appendage transcatheter occlusion to prevent stroke in high-risk patients with atrial fibrillation: early clinical experience. Circulation 2002; 105: 1887–9.

19. Nakai T, Lesh MD, Gerstenfeld EP, et al. Percutaneous left atrial appendage occlusion (PLAATO) for preventing cardioembolism: first experience in canine model. Circulation 2002; 105: 2217–22.

20. Veinot JP, Harrity PJ, Gentile F, et al. Anatomy of the normal left atrial appendage: a quantitative study of age-related changes in 500 autopsy hearts: implications for echocardiographic examination. Circulation 1997; 96: 3112–15.

21. Ernst G, Stollberger C, Abzieher F, et al. Morphology of the left atrial appendage. Anat Rec 1995; 242: 553–61.

22. Al-Saady NM, Obel OA, Camm AJ. Left atrial appendage: structure, function, and role in thromboembolism. Heart 1999; 82: 547–54.

23. Shirani J, Alaeddini J. Structural remodeling of the left atrial appendage in patients with chronic non-valvular atrial fibrillation: implications for thrombus formation, systemic embolism, and assessment by transesophageal echocardiography. Cardiovasc Pathol 2000; 9: 95–101.

24. Yu WC, Lee SH, Tai CT, et al. Reversal of atrial electrical remodeling following cardioversion of long-standing atrial fibrillation in man. Cardiovasc Res 1999; 42: 470–6.

25. Manning WJ. Role of transesophageal echocardiography in the management of thromboembolic stroke. Am J Cardiol 1997; 80: 19D–28D; discussion 35D–39D.

26. Li YH, Hwang JJ, Lin JL, et al. Importance of left atrial appendage function as a risk factor for systemic thromboembolism in patients with rheumatic mitral valve disease. Am J Cardiol 1996; 78: 844–7.

27. Pozzoli M, Febo O, Torbicki A, et al. Left atrial appendage dysfunction: a cause of thrombosis? Evidence by transesophageal echocardiography–Doppler studies. J Am Soc Echocardiogr 1991; 4: 435–41.

28. Neilson GH, Galea EG, Hossack KF. Thromboembolic complications of mitral valve disease. Aust N Z J Med 1978; 8: 372–6.

29. Rubin DN, Katz SE, Riley MF, et al. Evaluation of left atrial appendage anatomy and function in recent-onset atrial fibrillation by transesophageal echocardiography. Am J Cardiol 1996; 78: 774–8.

30. Tabata T, Oki T, Yamada H, et al. Role of left atrial appendage in left atrial reservoir function as evaluated by left atrial appendage clamping during cardiac surgery. Am J Cardiol 1998; 81: 327–32.

31. Nakamura M, Niinuma H, Chiba M, et al. Effect of the maze procedure for atrial fibrillation on atrial and brain natriuretic peptide. Am J Cardiol 1997; 79: 966–70.

32. Yoshihara F, Nishikimi T, Kosakai Y, et al. Atrial natriuretic peptide secretion and body fluid balance after bilateral atrial appendectomy by the maze procedure. J Thorac Cardiovasc Surg 1998; 116: 213–19.

33. Agmon Y, Khandheria BK, Gentile F, Seward JB. Echocardiographic assessment of the left atrial appendage. J Am Coll Cardiol 1999; 34: 1867–77.

34. Mikael Kortz RA, Delemarre BJ, van Dantzig JM, et al. Left atrial appendage blood flow determined by transesophageal echocardiography in healthy subjects. Am J Cardiol 1993; 71: 976–81.

35. Fukuchi M, Watanabe J, Kumagai K, et al. Increased von Willebrand factor in the endocardium as a local predisposing factor for thrombogenesis in overloaded human atrial appendage. J Am Coll Cardiol 2001; 37: 1436–42.

Chapter 8 Intracardiac echocardiography: transseptal catheterization

Walid Saliba, Jennifer E Cummings, Gery Tomassoni, and Andrea Natale

INTRODUCTION

Left atrial (LA) catheterization via the interatrial septum (IAS) has become a required skill for both electrophysiologists and interventional cardiologists. Transseptal puncture has been traditionally performed with the use of fluoroscopy. Intracardiac echocardiography (ICE)-guided transseptal catheterization has contributed to the effectiveness and, most importantly, the safety of this procedure. This is mainly related to several factors:

- it helps delineate the intracardiac anatomy, mainly the right and left atrial sizes
- it helps visualize the interatrial septum and some of the related anatomic variations and devices – thick, aneurysmal, parachute, patent foramen ovale (PFO), atrial septal defect (ASD), double patch, other repair devices
- it helps delineate the relation of the IAS to the anterior aorta and its posterior extension
- it helps visualize the area of the fossa ovalis, which is the thinnest part of the IAS
- it helps to determine the exact position of the tip of the transseptal sheath along the IAS and assess for tenting of the fossa ovalis by the dilator tip
- it helps confirm transseptal LA access via injection of saline (bubbles)
- it helps early recognition (therefore early intervention) of potential complications.

PROCEDURE

Vascular access is obtained via the femoral vein. The ICE catheter is advanced to the level of the right atrium (RA) in the "home view" position. Initial sweep is performed to identify the general intracardiac anatomy – in particular to evaluate the IAS for any anomalies. These include, among others, thick septum (lipomatous hypertrophy) (Figure 8.1), particularly after mitral valve (MV) or ASD repair, aneurysmal septum (Figure 8.2), double septum, probably secondary to persistence of the septum primum (Figure 8.3), PFO, ASD, and other closure devices.

An 8F transseptal sheath and dilator are then advanced over a 0.032 inch guidewire up to the level of the superior vena cava (SVC). The guidewire is exchanged with the Brockenbrough needle (BN), which is then loaded into the transseptal dilator and advanced to within 2 cm from the dilator tip. One might opt to leave the prepackaged inner stylet in the needle to protect the sheath from being scraped during the advancement of the needle. This can be removed when the needle is within the desired distance from the dilator tip. The Brockenbrough needle and the dilator/transseptal sheath assembly are then rotated toward the atrial septum, using the BN arrow as a guide to point toward the 3–6 o'clock position relative to its shaft. This assembly is then withdrawn slowly down to the level of the IAS under fluoroscopic guidance in the left anterior oblique (LAO) view. Although it is possible to track that withdrawal movement of the needle with ICE, it is recommended to leave the ICE catheter in the RA at the level of the IAS and use fluoroscopy during this brief withdrawal process. Pulling down from the high SVC location, the initial lateral movement of the tip of the needle coincides with the tip passing under the aortic knob. The second and more pronounced lateral movement occurs as the tip drops from the thick muscular IAS onto the thin fossa membrane. In this position, tenting of the IAS should be noted (Figure 8.4). Although this is true in most cases, two variables are important to optimize

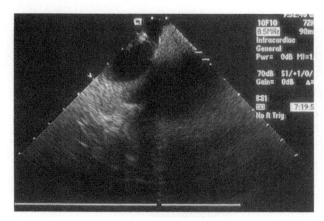

Figure 8.1 *An example of thick intratrial septum (IAS). RA = right atrium; LA = left atrium.*

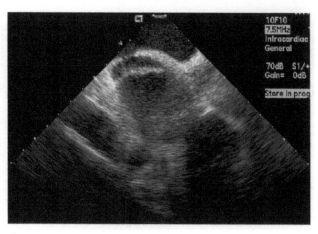

a

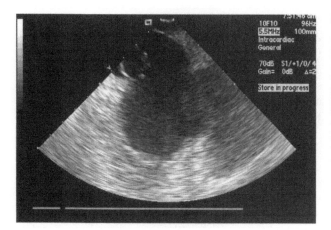

a

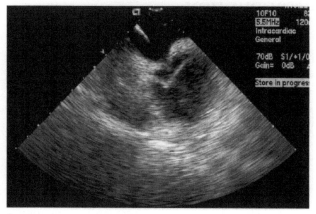

b

Figure 8.3 *(a) An example of a double septum, probably secondary to persistence of the septum premum. (b) An example of a transseptal puncture of a double septum. Note the "tenting".*

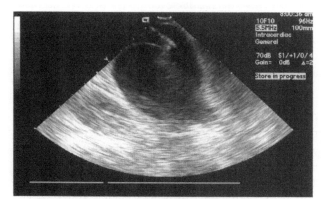

b

Figure 8.2 *(a) A septal aneurysm. By echocardiographic standards, an interatrial septal aneurysm is diagnosed when the excursion of the septum is more than 10 mm. (b) An example of a transseptal puncture in a patient with a septal aneurysm. In such cases, the transseptal needle can push the septum in the proximity of the opposite left atrial wall.*

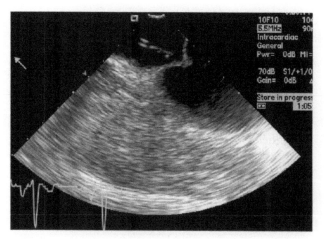

Figure 8.4 *During the transseptal puncture, note the deflection of the interatrial septum caused by the pressure of the needle "tenting".*

the transseptal puncture for the intended procedure: desired puncture site and minor anatomic variation (cardiac rotation).

The desired puncture site depends on the procedure to be performed. For example, for accessory pathways or MV procedure where access to the MV annulus is desired, the preferred puncture site would be slightly anterior. The ICE catheter can be positioned to visualize the IAS and the left atrial appendage (LAA) in the same plane and the dilator assembly can be rotated so as to confirm tenting in this specific plane; whereas, for procedures requiring reach to the pulmonary vein (PV) and posterior wall, a more posterior puncture is preferred to facilitate access to the right PVs. In this situation, the ICE catheter is rotated to visualize the IAS and the left PVs in the same plane and the dilator assembly can be rotated to confirm tenting in that plane. In some situations, the heart is slightly rotated and the initial needle orientation might not coincide exactly with the preferred puncture site at the level of the IAS. Therefore, continuous monitoring with ICE to localize the position of the tip of the dilator relative to the desired puncture site is recommended.

When visualizing the IAS, counterclockwise rotation of the ICE catheter will visualize anterior structures such as the aortic root (MV and LAA). Clockwise rotation will visualize posterior structures, such as a short-axis view of the antrum of the right pulmonary vein (RPV). In some difficult situations, using minor movement of the ICE catheter (rotating the ICE catheter one way or another, slight advancement and withdrawal of the catheter), one can localize the position of the dilator tip and guide it to the preferred puncture site. It is important to confirm that the dilator tip is in intimate contact and tenting at the preferred puncture site of the IAS before advancing the BN. The BN is then advanced slowly. During this process, it is important to monitor the position of the dilator tip, as the stiffness of the needle can displace the dilator superiorly toward the aorta or muscular ridge of the IAS. This occurs infrequently, but when it does, repositioning of the dilator should be performed and, occasionally, additional curvature is made on the BN, especially in cases with severe RA dilatation. One needs to make sure that tenting is not occurring at the level of the aortic root anteriorly (Figure 8.5), or too posteriorly at the level of the RA/LA recess. As the needle is advanced, tenting is accentuated. In some situations such as aneurysmal or double septum (Figure 8.2b), the distance from the tented fossa to the lateral LA wall is small. Reorientation of the dilator tip to maximize that space (usually more

anteriorly) should be done to minimize the risk of perforation.

The needle is then advanced through the septal membrane. During this process, a palpable pop is felt and a sudden "untenting" is confirmed by ICE. Injection of a small amount of saline (0.5 ml) via the needle and visualization of the bubbles in the LA confirms puncture of the septum and access to the LA (Figure 8.6). While keeping the needle position fixed, the dilator/sheath assembly is advanced 1–2 cm over the needle into the body of the LA. If the distance between the needle tip and the lateral wall of the LA is small, especially with more posterior puncture sites, it is recommended to rotate the needle anteriorly once in the LA to allow for more space and safety

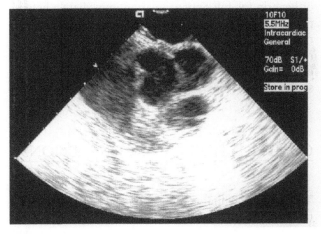

Figure 8.5 *The transseptal needle tenting at the level of the aortic root (canine).*

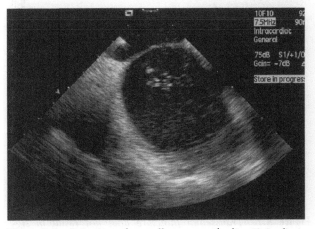

Figure 8.6 *Injection of a small amount of saline (0.5 ml) via the needle and visualization of the bubbles in the left atrium confirms successful puncture of the septum and access to the left atrium.*

to advance the dilator while maintaining the desired posterior puncture site. On some occasions, the IAS is stiff and advancement of the dilator might result in tenting of the IAS over the needle in the LA, which results in the needle falling back on the right side. In this situation, more advancement of the needle into the LA under ICE guidance can be done to provide the rail and stiffness for the dilator to be advanced into the LA. The dilator is then stabilized and the sheath advanced over the dilator and positioned anteriorly at the level of the MV annulus. In some situations, the needle can be advanced to but not beyond the tip of the dilator to provide the required stiffness to push it through a thick septum. The needle and dilator are then removed slowly to minimize the risk of air embolism and the sheath flushed appropriately. We recommend administration of heparin for full anticoagulation immediately before performing the transseptal puncture to minimize the risk of clot formation. Transseptal puncture does not result in significant interatrial shunting. Examination of such flow at the level of transseptal puncture is shown (Figure 8.8).

COMPLICATIONS AND CONCLUSIONS

The major potential complications related to transseptal puncture include:

- cardiac perforation resulting in tamponade (Figure 8.9)

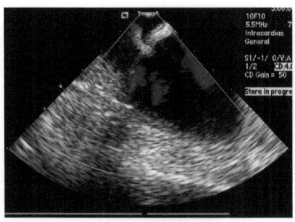

Figure 8.7 *Transseptal puncture does not result in significant interatrial shunting. A Doppler flow image reveals little interatrial shunting after removal of the transseptal sheath.*

- injury to other cardiac structures (aorta) (Figure 8.9)
- air embolization
- thromboembolic complication.

These can be minimized by confirming proper positioning of the dilator tip over the desired puncture site prior to advancing the needle and by monitoring the position of the dilator tip using ICE as the needle and the dilator/sheath assembly is advanced into the LA. Use of full heparinization shortly before the transseptal puncture reduces the risk of thromboembolization. To minimize air

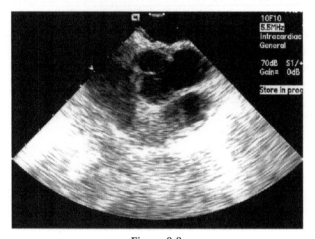

Figure 8.8

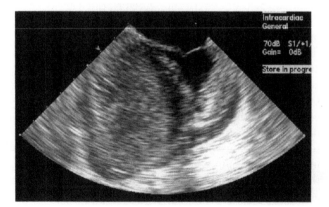

Figure 8.9

Figures 8.8 and 8.9 *Complications related to transseptal puncture. Figure 8.8 shows the transseptal needle at the aortic root secondary to an anterior puncture (canine). Figure 8.9 shows pericardial effusion secondary to perforation at the roof during transseptal puncture.*

embolization, removal of the catheters or dilator from the TS sheath should be done slowly, so as to avoid the air sucking effect, and adequate flushing of the sheaths after aspiration of all the air should be done prior to catheter insertion.

In conclusion, ICE is proving to be an important tool for transseptal access to the LA. By direct visualization of the puncture site and by early detection of potential complications, the safety and effectiveness of this procedure are optimized.

Chapter 9   **Right atrium: ICE in anatomic definition, mapping and ablation**

Richard J Hillock, Joseph B Morton, and Jonathan M Kalman

INTRODUCTION

Right atrial arrhythmias are the most common supraventricular arrhythmias treated by interventional electrophysiologists. The placement of electrophysiology catheters relies on an assumption that the patient has essentially normal atrial anatomy, and recognition of familiar electrographic signals as standard biplane fluoroscopy provides limited information on intracardiac structure. However, structures such as the crista terminalis, triangle of Koch, interatrial septum, Thebesian valve, and sub-Eustachian pouch have no direct fluoroscopic landmarks and have clinically important individual variation. These structures may give rise to tachyarrhythmias and are important landmarks for the interventional electrophysiologist. In addition, fluoroscopy is poor for monitoring complications of procedures. Radiographic cardiac silhouettes provide late information on perforation and pericardial collection and no information on lesion formation or minor catheter movement during ablation. Intracardiac echocardiography (ICE) allows definitive visualization of these endocardial structures, allows monitoring of potential complications, and facilitates direct and accurate catheter placement while ensuring good contact.

The two major platforms of intracardiac echocardiography are phased-array and mechanical transducers. The phased-array catheter is a 64-element array with a longitudinal imaging plane, with imaging frequencies of 5.5–10 MHz (depending on the imaging platform used). Imaging modalities include standard two-dimensional (2D), color wave, pulsed-wave, continuous-wave, and tissue Doppler imaging.[1,2] Mechanical transducer catheters utilize a 9 MHz crystal and present a 360° picture with the catheter in the center, familiar to users of intravascular ultrasound (IVUS), and uses the same imaging platform as IVUS (Boston Scientific Instruments). Depth of penetration is limited to 5 cm and, therefore, is the most useful for right atrial imaging alone.[3] In addition, recent developments in 3D ICE may allow reconstruction of RA anatomy with the ability to overlay intracardiac electrographic signals in an electro-anatomic approach similar to CARTO or Ensite.[4]

OVERVIEW OF RIGHT ATRIAL ANATOMY FOR THE ELECTROPHYSIOLOGIST

During embryologic development, the adult right atrium (RA) is derived from the primary right atrium, venous components, appendage, and vestibule (originating from the ventricular muscular tube).[5] The primary atrium forms the medial wall and the interatrial septum, the vascular part forms the posterior atrium between the cavae, the trabeculated atrial appendage forms the anterior roof, and the vestibule is the boundary between the pectinate atrium and the anteriorly placed tricuspid valve (Figure 9.1). The crista terminalis (CT), or terminal crest, is a cord-like structure that forms the boundary between the smooth venous component and the trabeculated atrium (Figure 9.2). The crista terminalis ramifies anteriorly into the pectinate right atrium and atrial appendage. The superior and medial end of the CT inserts into the region of the interatrial septum in close proximity to the insertion of Bachmann's bundle, while the inferior extent becomes continuous with the

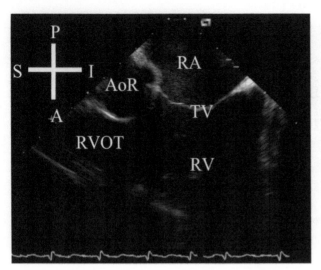

Figure 9.1 *Phased-array baseline image of the right atrium (RA). The transducer is vertical in the posterior RA, with the array pointing anteriorly. The right ventricle (RV) is seen clearly through the tricuspid valve (TV), the aortic root (AoR) is seen superiorly, with the right ventricular outflow tract (RVOT) anterior to the aortic root.*

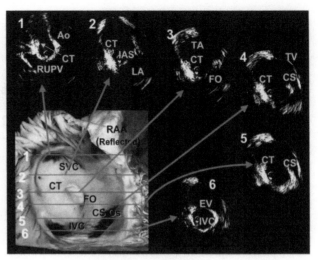

Figure 9.2 *Mechanical transducer images of the right atrium. The images are numbered sequentially from superior to inferior in the right atrium, with the anatomic correlation shown. (1) The high right atrium inferior to the superior vena cava (SVC) shows the relationship of the aorta (Ao), the right upper pulmonary vein (RUPV) to the crista terminalis (CT). (2) The level of the interatrial septum (IAS) with the left atrium (LA) seen poorly beyond, and the continuation of the CT. (3) The superior margin of the tricuspid annulus (TA) is seen anteriorly, and the fossa ovalis (FO) inferior to the IAS. (4 and 5) Continuing inferiorly brings the tricuspid valve (TV) into view and shows its relationship to the lateral CT, and medial coronary sinus (CS). (6) At the right atrial inferior vena cava (IVC) junction, the Eustachian valve is clearly seen marking the posterior rim of the inferior TA isthmus RAA = right atrial appendage. Reproduced with permission from Kalman JM et al.[12]*

Eustachian ridge and sends trabeculated ramifications into the isthmus.[6] The sinoatrial node is found within the CT at the level of the right atrium–superior vena cava (RA–SVC) junction and is a predominantly epicardial structure averaging 13–14 mm long.[7] The triangle of Koch is formed by the tendon of Todaro (an extension of the Eustachian valve) posteriorly, the hinge line of the septal leaflet of the tricuspid valve anteriorly, the coronary sinus (CS) os inferiorly, and the membranous atria-ventricular septum and penetrating bundle of His superiorly. The CS os may have a Thebesian valve that is sometimes muscular, usually fenestrated, and rarely imperforate.[6] In several elegant anatomic papers, Cabrera and co-workers have described the anatomy of the cavotricuspid isthmus (CTI). They described the region as a quadrilateral structure bounded by the tricuspid valve anteriorly, the Eustachian valve and inferior vena cava (IVC) posteriorly, the CS os septally, and the insertion of the crista terminalis laterally.[8] More recently, Cabrera et al provided a more detailed description of the anatomy of this region. They divided the isthmus into paraseptal (septal), inferior (mid), and inferolateral regions. Within each region are three morphologic sectors: the anterior smooth myocardial vestibule or pretricuspid region, the middle trabeculated sector, and the posterior membranous sector adjacent to the Eustachian valve. The paraseptal isthmus is in the region between the CS os and the septal leaflet of the tricuspid valve and has the thickest musculature.

The inferior or middle of the isthmus has the shortest distance from annulus to IVC and the least muscular of the divisions but contains the sub-Eustachian pouch. The lateral isthmus is more trabeculated and was the longest region of the isthmus.[6,9] The pouch is predominantly membranous, but up to 37% may have muscular fibers.[10] The anterior or vestibular region of the isthmus is predominantly muscular, with less muscle and more fibrofatty tissue seen in the posterior membranous area. However, anatomy in the isthmus can be highly variable.

The true interatrial septum is a small membranous ligament surrounded by muscular septum, superiorly bounded by the SVC and interatrial infolding, inferiorly by IVC, anteriorly by the triangle of Koch and the aortic root, and posteriorly by the RA wall and the pericardial space.[5,11]

SPECIFIC VISUALIZATION OF RIGHT ATRIAL STRUCTURES COMMONLY ASSOCIATED WITH TACHYCARDIA

THE SINOATRIAL NODE REGION AND CRISTA TERMINALIS

CT tachycardias account for approximately half to two-thirds of focal atrial tachycardias originating from within the RA.[12] Tachycardias may arise from along the length of this structure, although they are most commonly found at the superior region. These tachycardias frequently have electrophysiologic characteristics suggesting "micro-re-entry", although others may be automatic in mechanism.[12]

Accurate anatomic localization of the CT may be difficult with fluoroscopy alone. When required, ICE can be used to ensure contact and correct positioning of a mapping catheter along the CT during electrophysiology study and ablation[12,13] to guide mapping along this structure (Figures 9.3 and 9.4). In addition, the tip of the ablation catheter may be readily recognized by its fan-shaped artifact (Figure 9.5). The crista terminalis is well-visualized both with mechanical and phased-array ICE. When using the mechanical probe, it is first positioned in the SVC and then slowly pulled back through the body of the RA to the IVC–RA junction. The crista can be followed throughout its length as a ridge between the posterior

smooth-walled atrium and the anterior trabeculated atrium. The ridge is most prominent in the upper third of the RA. Superiorly, the ridge passes anterior to the SVC and inserts in the region of the superior interatrial septum. Inferiorly, it becomes continuous with the Eustachian ridge anterior to the IVC (Figure 9.6). When using phased-array ICE, the probe is placed in the posterior high RA, below the RA–SVC junction, and rotated towards the right atrial appendage (RAA) anteriorly. By sweeping the probe from medial to lateral (3 o'clock to 9 o'clock counterclockwise), the CT can be followed along its course between the smooth and trabeculated RA.

In the small proportion of patients with inappropriate sinus tachycardia who come to sinus node modification, the use of ICE is helpful in identifying the superior aspect of the CT and during ablation to monitor for the development of SVC stenosis, which has been described.[14,15]

CAVOTRICUSPID ISTHMUS IN CAVOTRICUSPID ISTHMUS-DEPENDENT ATRIAL FLUTTER

The CTI is well visualized by phased-array ICE during ablation of typical atrial flutter (Figure 9.7). While radiofrequency ablation (RFA) for the creation of a bidirectional conduction block across the isthmus has become first-line therapy in the management of typical CTI-dependent atrial flutter, the complex and variable anatomy of this region may be an impediment to achieving isthmus block. Cabrera and co-workers[8] have reported a wide range of anatomic variations within the isthmus, including pouches, recesses, trabeculations, and ridges, which may make successful ablation difficult (Figure 9.8). Large-tip and irrigated catheters facilitate isthmus ablation, but there is still a potential role for a real-time imaging modality which has the capability to accurately define CTI anatomy and guide RFA in difficult cases. Mechanical ICE has facilitated detailed endocardial mapping of the boundaries to the atrial flutter (AFL) isthmus[16,17] but is limited in its discrimination of other CTI features.[18] RA angiography may also give a general guide to CTI anatomy[19] but does not provide detailed endocardial definition or information regarding the thickness of the isthmus.

Recently, Morton et al used phased-array ICE with a high imaging frequency of between 7.5 MHz and 10 MHz in 15 patients undergoing ablation of typical AFL.[9] With this modality they were able to perform detailed analysis of the CTI in all patients (Figure 9.9). With the probe at the mid-atrial level, anteflex the

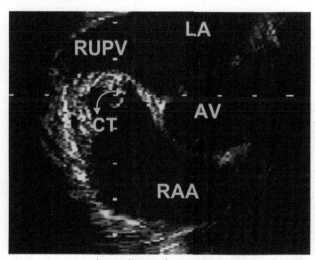

Figure 9.3 *Mechanical transducer ICE showing the relationships of the upper right atrium (crista terminalis (CT) and right atrial appendage (RAA)) to the right upper pulmonary vein (RUPV), aortic valve (AV), and left atrium (LA). In particular, the proximity of the superior CT to the RUPV is demonstrated. Reproduced with permission from Kalman JM et al.[12]*

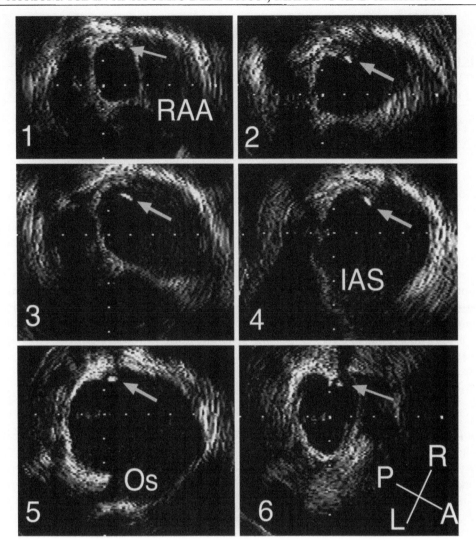

Figure 9.4 *Mechanical transducer images of a 20-pole electrophysiology catheter in place at the crista terminalis (CT). The close position of the catheter to the CT is evident throughout its length arrows. The images are sequential from superior to inferior in the right atrium, with the ICE catheter in the center of the image, and the lateral right atrium at the top of the picture. (1) Distal end of the crista catheter in the superior vena cava (SVC), (2)-(3) superior right atrium, (4) the level of the interatrial septum (IAS), (5) the level of the coronary sinus os (Os), and (6) the RA/IVC junction. (axis; P-posterior, A-anterior, R-right, L-left).*

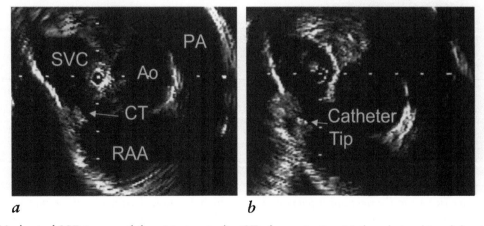

Figure 9.5 *Mechanical ICE images of the crista terminalis (CT) demonstrating (a) the relationship of the ridge-like CT to other right atrial structures, and (b) the accurate positioning of an electrophysiology catheter (Catheter Tip) during the ablation of a focal atrial tachycardia arising from the superior CT. The fan-shaped artifact from the tip of the ablation catheter is evident at the region of the superior and lateral CT. SVC = superior vena cava; Ao = aorta; PA = pulmonary artery; RAA = right atrial appendage. Reproduced with permission from Kalman JM et al.[15]*

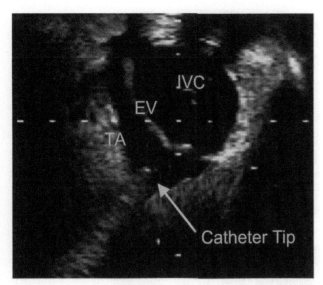

Figure 9.6 *Mechanical ICE image of ablation catheter placement during ablation of typical atrial flutter. A prominent Eustachian valve (EV) is seen with the ablation catheter (Catheter Tip) placed across the isthmus into the vestibular anterior isthmus (IVC = inferior vena cava; TA = tricuspid annulus). Although the gross anatomic landmarks of the isthmus can be demonstrated, the detail of the architecture cannot be seen with this technique.*

multiplane probe to visualize the inferior isthmus. Rotation of the catheter allows visualization of the isthmus from septal to lateral border. By removing the anteflexion at the lateral margin, the lateral annulus can be seen. The mechanical transducer is positioned at the level of the IVC–RA junction to visualize the Eustachian valve and ridge, and is then advanced to follow the anterior reach of the isthmus. The boundaries of the CTI (tricuspid annulus, Eustachian ridge, coronary sinus, and trabeculated free wall of the RA) were well-visualized in this study, as was the endocardial contour and shape, the presence of pouching, recesses and trabeculations, and the isthmus thickness along its length pre- and postablation. The thickness of the CTI measured as follows: anterior CTI (at the tricuspid annulus) = 4.1 ± 0.8 mm; mid CTI = 3.3 ± 0.5 mm; and posterior CTI (at the Eustachian ridge) = 2.7 ± 0.9 mm ($p < 0.001$ by ANOVA).

ICE was used to identify the ablation catheter and guide lesion delivery away from deep recesses and prominent trabeculations. Following each RFA application, a discrete lesion was usually visible, although this was more prominent when an 8-mm-tip RFA catheter was used. Over time (minutes) these lesions lost their definition and were replaced by a diffuse swelling of the CTI. Pouching and recesses were commonly seen and were usually deeper in the

septal rather than the lateral isthmus. In this study, ICE confirmed a long-held clinical impression: that there may be no single ideal anatomically determined location in the CTI to perform ablation. Although the septal isthmus is narrower in most patients, it is significantly more pouched. The location of thick trabeculae is variable throughout the CTI, but more frequently observed in the lateral isthmus.

The tricuspid annulus may be difficult to map and ensure good apposition to the annulus during ablation of right-sided accessory atrioventricular (AV) connections and tricuspid annular focal atrial tachycardia because the tricuspid annulus (TA) is a broad and highly mobile structure. ICE has been used to map the insertion of an AV bypass tract along the TA, while ensuring stable position and contact on the annulus.[20]

CORONARY SINUS OS AND TRIANGLE OF KOCH IN ATRIOVENTRICULAR NODAL RE-ENTRY TACHYCARDIA

The anatomy of the coronary sinus ostium may be highly variable and this has implications for ablation of atrioventricular nodal re-entry tachycardia (AVNRT). Delurgio et al used IAC to evaluate posteroseptal space anatomy in patients with atrioventricular nodal re-entrant tachycardia compared with patients with other mechanisms of tachycardia. The posteroseptal space was found to be significantly wider in patients with atrioventricular nodal re-entry tachycardia, suggesting an anatomic basis for dual atrioventricular nodal physiology.[21] Fisher et al used ICE to guide slow-pathway ablation in patients with AVNRT.[22] They observed that ablation at the tricuspid valve's insertion into the AV muscular septum, as identified by ICE, reliably terminated anterograde slow-pathway conduction, supporting the hypothesis that the slow pathway consistently traverses this anatomic location.

OTHER RIGHT ATRIAL APPLICATIONS OF INTRACARDIAC ECHOCARDIOGRAPHY

FOSSA OVALIS AND TRANSSEPTAL PUNCTURE

Transseptal puncture is a standard approach to the left atrium. Commonly, the transseptal puncture is performed under fluoroscopic guidance with or without the assistance of transesophageal echocardiography. ICE allows accurate and real-time evaluation of the

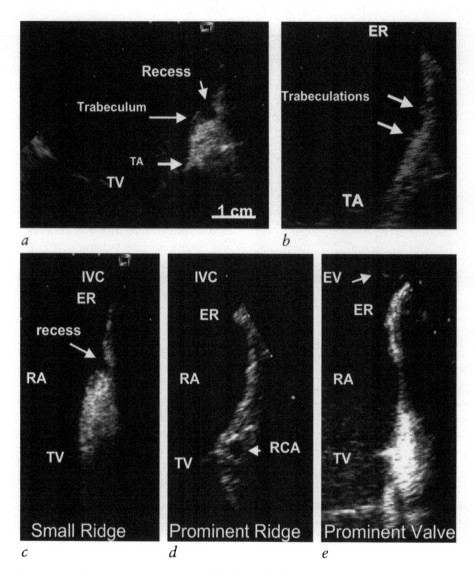

Figure 9.7 *Significant normal variation of cavotricuspid isthmus (CTI) seen on phased-array ICE. The isthmus may have trabeculations, recesses or crypts (a,b), prominent Eustachian ridges (ER) (c,d), and a Eustachian valve (EV), as shown (e). Visualization of these variations may allow accurate placement of CTI linear ablation to affect a line of block in ablation of CTI-dependent atrial flutter. RA = right atrium; TA = tricuspid annulus; TV = tricuspid valve; IVC = inferior vena cava; RCA = right coronary artery. Reproduced with permission from Morton JB et al.[9]*

stages of transseptal puncture without significantly impeding the fluoroscopic field and gives detailed information on adjacent structures without requiring general anesthesia. The efficacy of this approach has been well demonstrated.[23–27] Both mechanical and phased-array systems are highly effective for this purpose (Figure 9.10).

COMPLEX CONGENITAL HEART DISEASE

Patients with complex surgical correction of congenital heart defects are at increased risk of atrial arrhythmias, typically relating to the associated atrial scarring.[28] Normal anatomy can also be distorted and may pose an increased risk of complications. ICE has been used to identify anatomy and guide catheter placement in a patient with baffle-related atrial flutter in corrected D-transposition of the great arteries.[29]

INTRAPROCEDURAL MONITORING

ICE has real-time applications in monitoring the development and placement of lesions, and early detection of complications. The pericardial space is

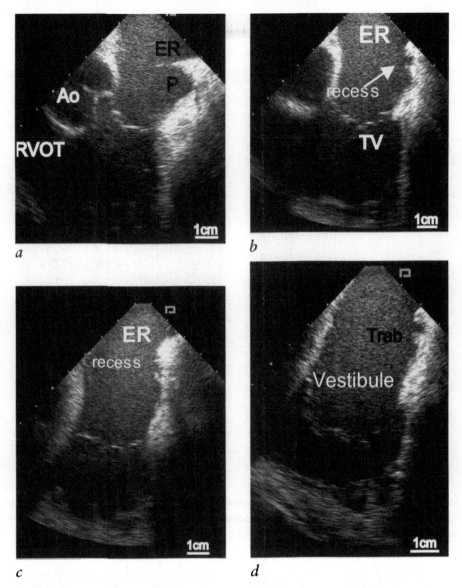

Figure 9.8 *Phased-array image of the cavotricuspid isthmus demonstrating the change in characteristics between the paraseptal isthmus and the lateral isthmus. (a) The septal isthmus: a prominent Eustachian ridge (ER) with a large sub-Eustachian pouch (P) is shown. (b,c) The mid isthmus shows a prominent ridge with a small recess and the smooth vestibular component of the isthmus. (d) Significant trabecular (Trab) ramifications of the distal crista terminalis (CT) in the lateral isthmus. Ao = aorta; RVOT = right ventricular outflow tract; TV = tricuspid valve. Reproduced with permission from Morton JB et al.[9]*

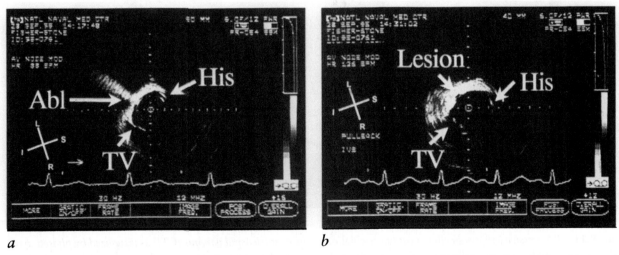

Figure 9.9 *Mechanical ICE images of atrioventricular nodal re-entrant tachycardia (AVNRT) ablation. (a) Pre-ablation: the ablation catheter tip (Ab1 and, fan-shaped artifact) overlying the muscular AV septum. (b) Post-ablation: the lesion is clearly seen. Reproduced with permission from Fisher et al.[22]*

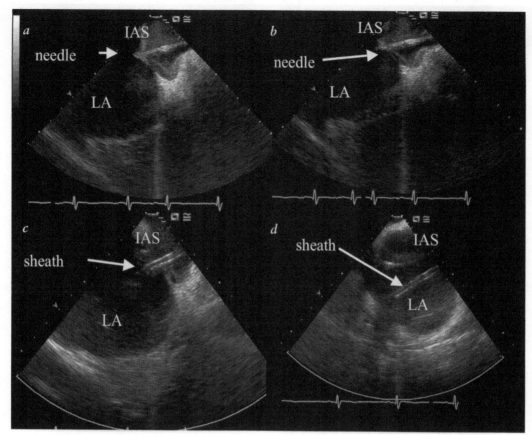

Figure 9.10   *Phased-array imaging of interatrial septal puncture. (a) Tenting of the interatrial septum (IAS) by the needle. (b) The moment of puncture by the needle. (c) The sheath is advanced into the left atrium (LA) through the puncture. (d) The transseptal sheath well within the left atrium.*

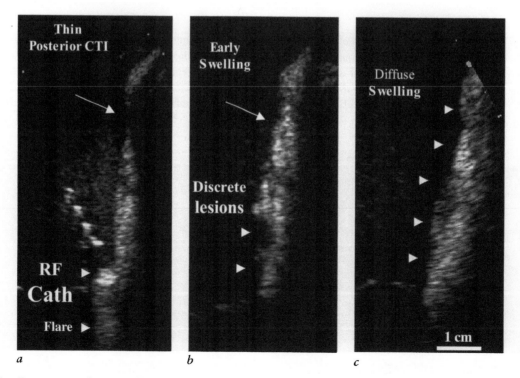

Figure 9.11   *Progressive isthmus swelling post linear ablation of the cavotricuspid isthmus (CTI) as visualized by phased-array ICE. (a) Onset radiofrequency ablation (RFA): the RF catheter is at the anterior margin of the inferior tricuspid isthmus. (b) Early post RFA: the formation of RF lesions seen as discrete lesions with the later development of confluent edema and swelling – post-RFA (c). Reproduced with permission from Morton et al.[9]*

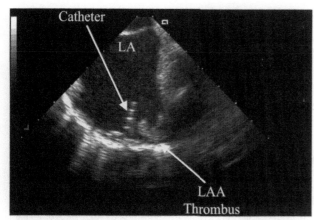

Figure 9.12 *Phased-array image of the development of thrombus associated with radiofrequency catheter ablation. This image is taken from an ablation in the left atrium (LA) with associated thrombus formation in the left atrial appendage (LAA). The ablation catheter and the thrombus are marked by arrows.*

easily visualized and the development of a pericardial collection can be demonstrated before the patient develops hemodynamic and fluoroscopic evidence of compromise. Lesion formation can be directly visualized and has been used to monitor radiofrequency[30] and cryotherapy delivery[31,32] (Figure 9.11). ICE allows the direct visualization and placement of linear ablations[33,34] and can be used to monitor for coagulum, overheating,[35] and thrombus (Figure 9.12). Catheter

contact and stability are confirmed when ICE is utilized during radiofrequency ablation and allow greater certainty that effective energy is delivered to the appropriate substrate.[32,36–38]

SUMMARY

Intracardiac echocardiography has provided critical insights into the role of right atrial anatomy in electrophysiology and helped to define the mechanism of a variety of arrhythmias. There are a number of benefits of direct endocardial visualization during RF ablation, including:

1. precise anatomic localization of the ablation catheter tip in relation to important endocardial structures that cannot be visualized with fluoroscopy
2. reduction in fluoroscopy time
3. evaluation of catheter-tip–tissue contact
4. confirmation of lesion formation and identification of lesion size and continuity
5. immediate identification of complications.

ICE is an excellent clinical and experimental research tool to help in understanding the critical role played by specific right atrial endocardial structures in arrhythmogenesis.

REFERENCES

1. Hynes BJ, Mart C, Artman S, et al. Role of intracardiac ultrasound in interventional electrophysiology. Curr Opin Cardiol 2004; 19: 52–7.
2. Siemens Medical. AcuNav Product Specifications, 2005. Internet communication.
3. Bruce CJ, Friedman PA. Intracardiac echocardiography. Eur J Echocardiogr 2001; 2: 234–44.
4. Rao L, He R, Ding C, et al. Novel noncontact catheter system for endocardial electrical and anatomical imaging. Ann Biomed Eng 2004; 32: 573–84.
5. Anderson RH, Brown NA, Webb S. Development and structure of the atrial septum. Heart 2002; 88: 104–10.
6. Ho SY, Anderson RH, Sanchez-Quintana D. Atrial structure and fibres: morphologic bases of atrial conduction. Cardiovasc Res 2002; 54: 325–36.
7. Sanchez-Quintana D, Cabrera JA, Farre J, et al. Sinus node revisited in the era of electroanatomical mapping and catheter ablation. Heart 2005; 91: 189–94.
8. Cabrera JA, Sanchez-Quintana D, Ho SY, et al. The architecture of the atrial musculature between the orifice of the inferior caval vein and the tricuspid valve: the anatomy of the isthmus. J Cardiovasc Electrophysiol 1998; 9: 1186–95.
9. Morton JB, Sanders P, Davidson NC, et al. Phased-array intracardiac echocardiography for defining cavotricuspid isthmus anatomy during radiofrequency ablation of typical atrial flutter. J Cardiovasc Electrophysiol 2003; 14: 591–7.
10. Cabrera JA, Sanchez-Quintana D, Farre J, et al. The inferior right atrial isthmus: further architectural insights for current and coming ablation technologies. J Cardiovasc Electrophysiol 2005; 16: 402–8.
11. Anderson RH, Webb S, Brown NA. Clinical anatomy of the atrial septum with reference to its developmental components. Clin Anat 1999; 12: 362–74.
12. Kalman JM, Olgin JE, Karch MR, et al. "Cristal tachycardias": origin of right atrial tachycardias from the crista terminalis identified by intracardiac echocardiography. J Am Coll Cardiol 1998; 31: 451–9.
13. Marchlinski FE, Ren JF, Schwartzman D, et al. Accuracy of fluoroscopic localization of the crista terminalis documented by intracardiac echocardiography. J Interv Card Electrophysiol 2000; 4: 415–21.
14. Lesh MD, Kalman JM, Karch MR. Use of intracardiac echocardiography during electrophysiologic evaluation and therapy of atrial arrhythmias. J Cardiovasc Electrophysiol 1998; 9: S40–S47.

15. Kalman JM, Lee RJ, Fisher WG, et al. Radiofrequency catheter modification of sinus pacemaker function guided by intracardiac echocardiography. Circulation 1995; 92: 3070–81.

16. Olgin JE, Kalman JM, Fitzpatrick AP, et al. Role of right atrial endocardial structures as barriers to conduction during human type I atrial flutter: activation and entrainment mapping guided by intracardiac echocardiography. Circulation 1995; 92: 1839–48.

17. Kalman JM, Olgin JE, Saxon LA, et al. Activation and entrainment mapping defines the tricuspid annulus as the anterior barrier in typical atrial flutter. Circulation 1996; 94: 398–406.

18. Darbar D, Olgin JE, Miller JM, et al. Localization of the origin of arrhythmias for ablation: from electrocardiography to advanced endocardial mapping systems. J Cardiovasc Electrophysiol 2001; 12: 1309–25.

19. Heidbuchel H, Willems R, van Rensburg H, et al. Right atrial angiographic evaluation of the posterior isthmus: relevance for ablation of typical atrial flutter. Circulation 2000; 101: 2178–84.

20. Ren JF, Schwartzman D, Callans DJ, et al. Intracardiac echocardiographic imaging in guiding and monitoring radiofrequency catheter ablation at the tricuspid annulus. Echocardiography 1998; 15: 661–4.

21. Delurgio DB, Frohwein SC, Walter PF, et al. Anatomy of atrioventricular nodal reentry investigated by intracardiac echocardiography. Am J Cardiol 1997; 80: 231–4.

22. Fisher WG, Pelini MA, Bacon ME. Adjunctive intracardiac echocardiography to guide slow pathway ablation in human atrioventricular nodal reentrant tachycardia: anatomic insights. Circulation 1997; 96: 3021–9.

23. Daoud EG, Kalbfleisch SJ, Hummel JD. Intracardiac echocardiography to guide transseptal left heart catheterization for radiofrequency ablation. J Cardiovasc Electrophysiol 1999; 10: 358–63.

24. Szili-Torok T, Kimman GP, Theuns D, et al. Transseptal left heart catheterization guided by intracardiac echocardiography. Heart 2001; 86: E11.

25. Citro R, Ducceschi V, Salustri A, et al. Intracardiac echocardiography to guide transseptal catheterization for radiofrequency catheter ablation of left-sided accessory pathways in humans: two case reports. Cardiovasc Ultrasound 2004; 2: 20.

26. Tardif JC, Vannan MA, Miller DS, et al. Potential applications of intracardiac echocardiography in interventional electrophysiology. Am Heart J 1994; 127: 1090–4.

27. Shalganov TN, Paprika D, Borbas S, et al. Preventing complicated transseptal puncture with intracardiac echocardiography: case report. Cardiovasc Ultrasound 2005; 3: 5.

28. Rhodes JF Jr, Qureshi AM, Preminger TJ, et al. Intracardiac echocardiography during transcatheter interventions for congenital heart disease. Am J Cardiol 2003; 92: 1482–4.

29. Kedia A, Hsu PY, Holmes J, et al. Use of intracardiac echocardiography in guiding radiofrequency catheter ablation of atrial tachycardia in a patient after the senning operation. Pacing Clin Electrophysiol 2003; 26: 2178–80.

30. Kalman JM, Jue J, Sudhir K, et al. In vitro quantification of radiofrequency ablation lesion size using intracardiac echocardiography in dogs. Am J Cardiol 1996; 77: 217–19.

31. Okishige K, Harada T, Kawabata M, et al. Transvenous catheter cryoablation of the atrioventricular node and visual assessment of freezing of cardiac tissue using intracardiac echocardiography. Jpn Heart J 2004; 45: 513–20.

32. Dubuc M, Khairy P, Rodriguez-Santiago A, et al. Catheter cryoablation of the atrioventricular node in patients with atrial fibrillation: a novel technology for ablation of cardiac arrhythmias. J Cardiovasc Electrophysiol 2001; 12: 439–44.

33. Olgin JE, Kalman JM, Chin M, et al. Electrophysiological effects of long, linear atrial lesions placed under intracardiac ultrasound guidance. Circulation 1997; 96: 2715–21.

34. Roithinger FX, Steiner PR, Goseki Y, et al. Low-power radiofrequency application and intracardiac echocardiography for creation of continuous left atrial linear lesions. J Cardiovasc Electrophysiol 1999; 10: 680–91.

35. Marrouche NF, Martin DO, Wazni O, et al. Phased-array intracardiac echocardiography monitoring during pulmonary vein isolation in patients with atrial fibrillation: impact on outcome and complications. Circulation 2003; 107: 2710–16.

36. Kalman JM, Fitzpatrick AP, Olgin JE, et al. Biophysical characteristics of radiofrequency lesion formation in vivo: dynamics of catheter tip–tissue contact evaluated by intracardiac echocardiography. Am Heart J 1997; 133: 8–18.

37. Chu E, Kalman JM, Kwasman MA, et al. Intracardiac echocardiography during radiofrequency catheter ablation of cardiac arrhythmias in humans. J Am Coll Cardiol 1994; 24: 1351–7.

38. Lee RJ, Kalman JM, Fitzpatrick AP, et al. Radiofrequency catheter modification of the sinus node for "inappropriate" sinus tachycardia. Circulation 1995; 92: 2919–28.

Chapter 10   Intracardiac echocardiography in the congenital catheterization laboratory

Piers CA Barker and John F Rhodes Jr

INTRODUCTION

Intracardiac echocardiography (ICE) represents the most recent step of an ongoing evolution towards better imaging for congenital heart disease, from fluoroscopy to transthoracic echocardiography, and from transesophageal to intracardiac echocardiography. Its distinction from intravascular ultrasound (IVUS) also parallels the development of increasingly sophisticated two-dimensional (2D) ultrasound imaging, with adequate frame rates in all modalities of use. The first human experience,[1] reported in 2002, introduced ICE as an important tool in the electrophysiology laboratory, with rapid acceptance for aiding in transseptal puncture of the atrial septum and pulmonary vein isolation procedures. Once its utility in creating an interatrial communication was demonstrated, it was a small step to use ICE for closing interatrial shunts, and its application to congenital heart disease began.

Since these first studies, ICE has been used for a progressively expanding number of diagnoses and interventional procedures in the congenital cardiac catheterization laboratory.[2,3] Its strengths include the probe's proximity to intracardiac structures, the absence of any air–tissue interference in the blood pool, and its maneuverability to achieve almost any orthogonal view. These strengths make it an ideal adjunct imaging tool in the congenital catheterization laboratory, as it permits more accurate assessment of the congenital heart defect and real-time guidance of intervention in combination with fluoroscopy. Limitations do remain, such as imaging of the left pulmonary artery, pulmonary valve, and aortic isthmus, but these are more related to the current probe size limiting aggressive manipulation. ICE can therefore be viewed as the cutting edge of an evolving paradigm, in which multiple imaging tools can be used to treat congenital heart disease, as the following examples will demonstrate.

PATENT FORAMEN OVALE

ANATOMY

The patent foramen ovale (PFO) is a normal structure in fetal life, formed by coalescing fenestrations in the septum primum creating an interatrial communication, bounded by the thicker septum secundum, with the remaining septum primum forming the flap valve on the left atrial side. After birth, the flap valve of septum primum is pushed against the septum secundum by the higher left atrial pressures, and eventually seals by 4–6 months of age.[4] However, in 25% of otherwise normal adults, the sealing of the flap valve is incomplete and potential separation of the flap valve from the septum secundum is possible, leaving the interatrial communication unguarded for right to left shunting.

Several variations on patent foramen ovale exist, and these are demonstrated below:

- Tunnel defect, in which there is considerable overlap of septum primum and septum secundum and limited movement of the flap valve:
  - PFO tunnel – open (Figure 10.1a)
  - PFO tunnel – closed (Figure 10.1b).
- Aneurysmal septum primum (atrial septum primum, ASA), in which there is a very redundant flap valve that may cross into the right atrium:
  - PFO – ASA (Figure 10.1c).
- Fenestrated septum primum, with multiple defects of varying size:
  - Fenestrated PFO – large defect (Figure 10.1d)
  - Fenestrated PFO – small defect (Figure 10.1e).

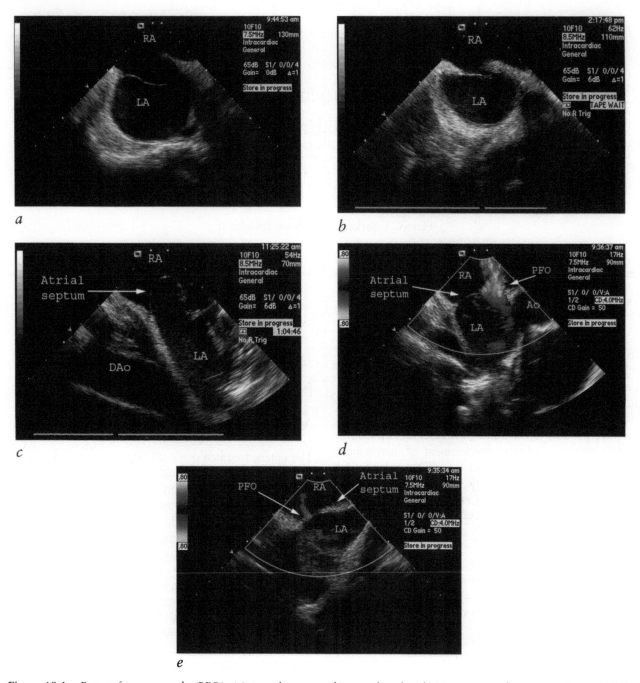

Figure 10.1 *Patent foramen ovale (PFO): (a) tunnel – open; (b) tunnel – closed; (c) aneurysmal septum primum (ASA); (d) fenestrated, large defect; (e) fenestrated, small defect. DAo = descending aorta; LA = left atrium; PFO = patent foramen ovale; RA = right atrium.*

COLOR DOPPLER AND AGITATED SALINE CONTRAST

The potential for right to left (R to L) shunting can be demonstrated during the ICE study by color Doppler and with right atrial injection of agitated saline contrast, both of which are demonstrated:

- Tunnel PFO – color – R to L (Figure 10.2a)
- Tunnel PFO – bubbles – R to L (Figure 10.2b).

Two of the currently available devices (CardioSEAL and Amplatzer) that are used for PFO closure are now considered.

CardioSEAL

- Left atrial (LA) disk deployment:
  - PFO – CardioSEAL – LA disk (Figure 10.3a).
- Right atrial (RA) disk deployment:
  - PFO – CardioSEAL – RA disk (Figure 10.3b).

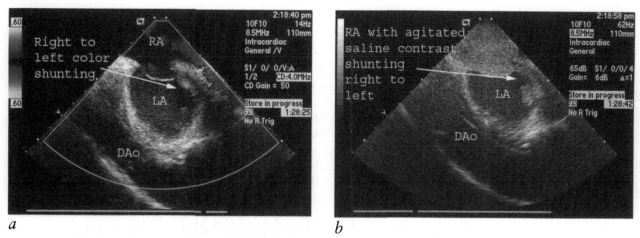

Figure 10.2 *Tunnel PFO: (a) color, R to L; (b) bubbles, R to L. DAo = descending aorta; LA = left atrium; RA = right atrium.*

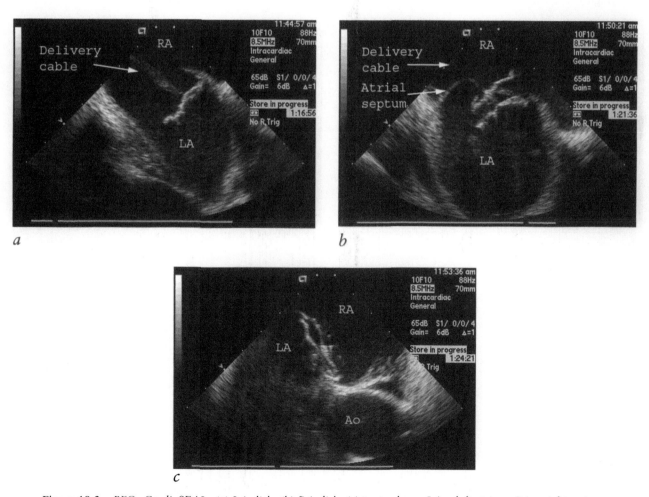

Figure 10.3 *PFO, CardioSEAL: (a) LA disk; (b) RA disk; (c) post release. LA = left atrium; RA = right atrium.*

- Final deployment:
  - PFO – CardioSEAL – post release (Figure 10.3c).

AMPLATZER

- LA disk deployment:
  - PFO – Amplatzer – LA disk (Figure 10.4a).
- RA disk deployment:
  - PFO – Amplatzer – RA disk (Figure 10.4b).
- Final deployment:
  - PFO – Amplatzer – post release (Figure 10.4c).

AGITATED SALINE CONTRAST

After device placement, elimination of the right to left shunt can be proven by repeat injection of agitated saline contrast directly through the delivery sheath:

- PFO – CardioSEAL – bubbles – post release (Figure 10.5a)
- PFO – Amplatzer – bubbles – post release (Figure 10.5b).

ATRIAL SEPTAL DEFECT

ANATOMY

Secundum atrial septal defects (ASDs) occur in the same location as patent foramen ovale (namely, the fossa ovalis), but with one crucial distinction: whereas in a PFO the flap valve of septum primum is adequate in size to cover the interatrial communication, in a true secundum ASD the flap valve is deficient or absent. This produces a persistent interatrial shunt, which is predominantly left to right as a result of the decreased left ventricular compliance and higher left ventricular diastolic pressures. With time, this leads to right heart volume overload, and the potential for later arrhythmias and pulmonary hypertension.[5,6]

Several variations on this anatomy also exist:

- Common secundum atrial septal defect:
  - ASD common secundum (Figure 10.6a).
- The resting diameter measurement, shown here, demonstrates the chronic nature of the interatrial shunt:
  - ASD – resting (Figure 10.6b).

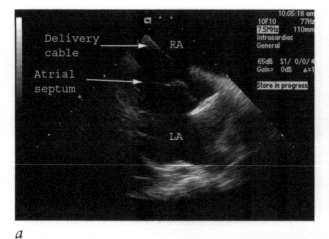

a

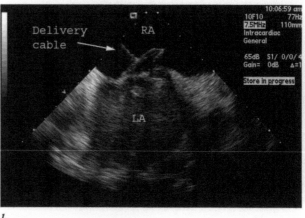

b

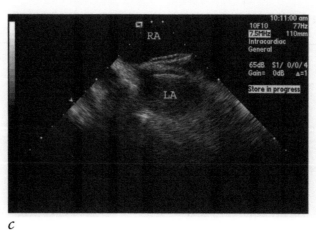

c

Figure 10.4 *PFO, Amplatzer: (a) LA disk; (b) RA disk; (c) post release. LA = left atrium; RA = right atrium.*

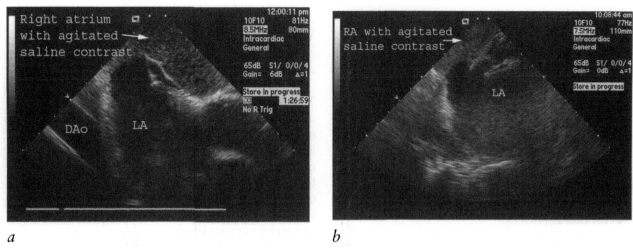

Figure 10.5   *PFO, bubbles: (a) CardioSEAL; (b) Amplatzer. LA = left atrium; RA = right atrium.*

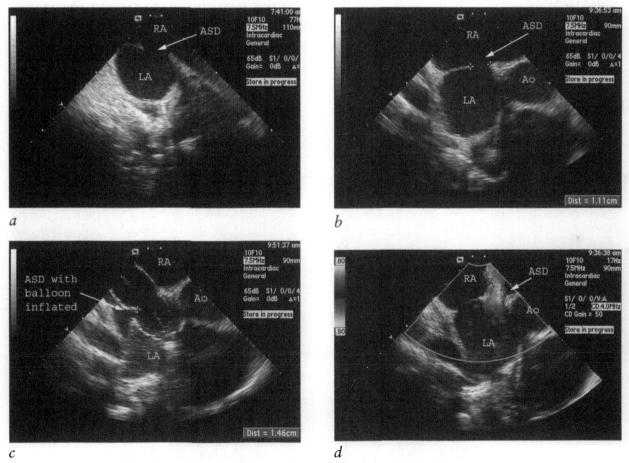

Figure 10.6   *Atrial septal defect (ASD): (a) common secundum; (b) resting; (c) stretch diameter; (d) color flow. Ao = Aorta; ASD = atrial septal defect; LA = left atrium; RA = right atrium.*

- The balloon stretch diameter demonstrates the limits of the defect, correlating with size of device needed to securely close the defect:
  - ASD – stretch diameter (Figure 10.6c).
- Color Doppler demonstrates the left to right direction of the shunt pre-intervention, as well as helps exclude fenestrated defects or defects

in other parts of the interatrial septum not amenable to catheter-based closure:
  - ASD – color flow (Figure 10.6d).

Similar to the experience with patent foramen ovale, several devices exist for atrial septal defect closure that are amenable to ICE guidance.

HELEX

- LA disk deployment:
    - HELEX LA disk (Figure 10.7a).
- RA disk deployment:
    - HELEX RA disk (Figure 10.7b).
- Final deployment:
    - HELEX deployed (Figure 10.7c).

AMPLATZER

- LA disk deployment:
    - Amplatzer ASD – LA disk (Figure 10.8a).
- RA disk deployment:
    - Amplatzer ASD – RA disk (Figure 10.8b).
- Final deployment:
    - Amplatzer ASD – deployed (Figure 10.8c).
- Color Doppler through device interstices:
    - Amplatzer ASD – deployed – color (Figure 10.8d).

SIDERIS TRANSCATHETER PATCH

- ASD – Sideris – balloon (Figure 10.9).

VENTRICULAR SEPTAL DEFECT

ANATOMY

The reported experience of using ICE for ventricular septal defects (VSDs) is small, mainly due to the ongoing trials of various VSD devices. Reported uses have therefore mainly consisted of adult patients with acquired muscular VSDs (post-myocardial infarction), although the ability of ICE to image the left ventricular outflow tract suggests utility for more basal defects involving the paramembranous septum.

PARAMEMBRANOUS VSD WITH SIDERIS DOUBLE BALLOON PATCH

- 2D anatomy of ventricular septal defect:
    - Paramembranous VSD – 2D (Figure 10.10a).
- Color flow of defect:
    - Paramembranous VSD – color (Figure 10.10b).
- Left ventricular (LV) balloon:
    - Paramembranous VSD – Sideris – LV balloon (Figure 10.10c).

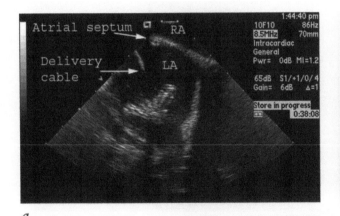

a

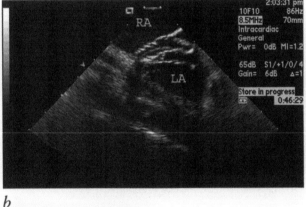

b

c

Figure 10.7 *Helex: (a) LA disk; (b) RA disk; (c) deployed. LA = left atrium; RA = right atrium.*

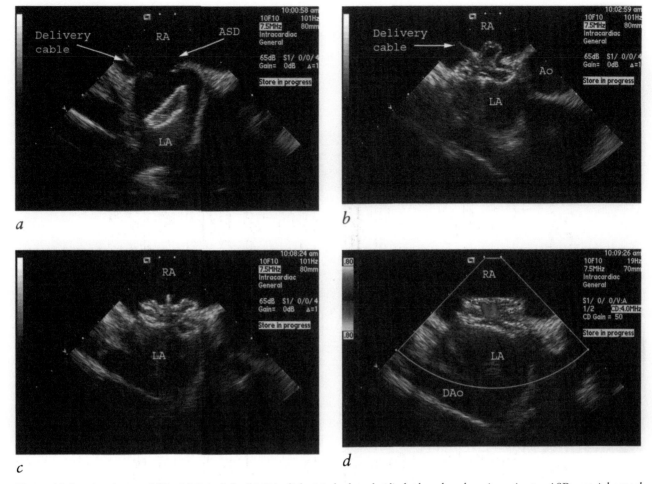

Figure 10.8   *Amplatzer, ASD: (a) LA disk; (b) RA disk; (c) deployed; (d) deployed, color. Ao = Aorta; ASD = atrial septal defect; DAo = descending aorta; LA = left atrium; RA = right atrium.*

- Right ventricular (RV) balloon:
  - Paramembranous VSD – Sideris – RV balloon (Figure 10.10d).

PULMONARY ARTERIOVENOUS MALFORMATIONS

ANATOMY

Pulmonary arteriovenous malformations (AVMs) may exist in the setting of congenital vascular syndromes, such as Osler–Weber–Rendu syndrome, other palliated forms of congenital heart disease, such as patients with only superior vena caval (SVC) flow to the pulmonary arteries (Glenn, bidirectional Glenn, hemi-Fontan, or Kawashima procedures), or may be acquired in the setting of hepatic cirrhosis or portocaval shunts. These can be mistaken for interatrial communications on transthoracic or transesophageal ultrasound, or may coexist with an ASD, making the recognition of this condition essential.

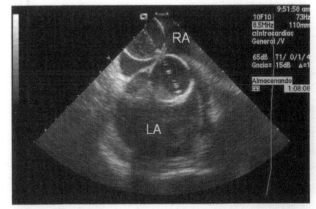

Figure 10.9   *ASD, Sideris, balloon. LA = left atrium; RA = right atrium.*

- Color flow of left pulmonary veins:
  - Pulm AVM – color (Figure 10.11a).
- Agitated saline injection with selective return to left lower pulmonary vein:
  - Pulm AVM – contrast (Figure 10.11b).

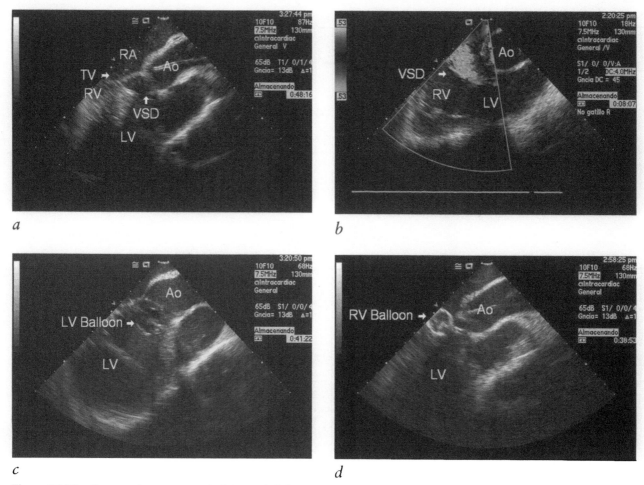

Figure 10.10 *Paramembranous ventricular septal deficit (VSD): (a) 2D; (b) color; (c) Sideris, LV balloon; (d) Sideris, RV balloon; Ao = Aorta; LV = left ventricle; RA = right atrium; RV = right ventricle; TV = tricuspid valve; VSD = ventricular septal deficit.*

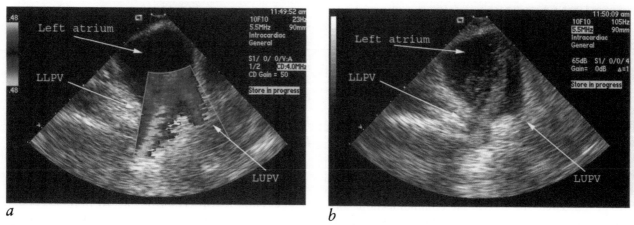

Figure 10.11 *Pulmonary arteriovenous malformations (AVM): (a) color; (b) contrast. LLPV = left lower pulmonary vein; LUPV = left upper pulmonary vein.*

PULMONARY VEIN STENOSIS

ANATOMY

Pulmonary vein stenosis can occur in many settings, from a rare primary congenital defect to an acquired lesion. Acquired pulmonary vein stenosis is often a complication of a procedure performed near the pulmonary venous ostium, such as an anastomosis for forms of anomalous pulmonary venous connection, or after radiofrequency ablation for pulmonary vein isolation. ICE imaging permits improved catheter positioning for balloon or stent procedures for these stenotic vessels, as well as providing immediate feedback on change in flow dynamics.

LEFT UPPER PULMONARY VEIN (LUPV) STENOSIS FOLLOWING RADIOFREQUENCY ABLATION

- Color Doppler of turbulent flow entering the left atrium:
  - LUPV color – preballoon (Figure 10.12a).
- Spectral Doppler tracing of left upper pulmonary vein flow pre-intervention:
  - LUPV Doppler – preballoon (Figure 10.12b).
- Spectral Doppler tracing of unobstructed right lower pulmonary vein (RLPV) for comparison:
  - RLPV Doppler – normal (Figure 10.12c).
- Balloon angioplasty of left upper pulmonary vein:
  - LUPV balloon (Figure 10.12d).
- Color Doppler post-angioplasty:
  - LUPV color – postballoon (Figure 10.12e).
- Spectral Doppler post-angioplasty:
  - LUPV Doppler – postballoon (Figure 10.12f).

RIGHT UPPER PULMONARY VEIN (RUPV) STENOSIS FOLLOWING SINUS VENOSUS ASD REPAIR

- 2D image of right pulmonary vein:
  - RUPV 2D (Figure 10.13a).
- Color Doppler of turbulent flow entering the left atrium:
  - RUPV – color – preballoon (Figure 10.13b).
- Balloon angioplasty of right pulmonary vein:
  - RUPV balloon (Figure 10.13c).
- Color Doppler post-angioplasty:
  - RUPV – color – postballoon (Figure 10.13d).

LEFT VENTRICULAR OUTFLOW TRACT DISEASE

ANATOMY

Left ventricular outflow tract disease is an example of a region outside the atria that is very amenable to ICE imaging and guidance of interventional procedures. This area can be imaged safely from the right atrium and falls into a mid-field imaging depth optimal for the current transducer sizes and frequencies. Additionally, imaging from the right atrium (for aortic valves) or positioning of the ICE probe in the low SVC (for supravalvar disease) permits real-time guidance of the interventional procedure without any risk of interfering with catheter position. The baseline anatomy, function, and annulus or vessel measurements can be fully assessed prior to intervention, and repeat functional assessment can be performed after intervention to permit correlation with follow-up transthoracic echocardiograms. Catheter position can also be guided to increase the accuracy of pressure measurements for stenoses in series. Conceivably, the use of ICE in this setting could decrease the need for angiography, thus eliminating dye exposure and reducing radiation dose to the patient.

AORTIC STENOSIS (AS)

- 2D anatomy, long-axis (LAX) view:
  - AS – LAX 2D (Figure 10.14a).
- 2D anatomy, short-axis view:
  - AS – valve – preballoon (Figure 10.14b).
- Left ventricular hypertrophy (LVH), diastole:
  - AS – LVH – diastole (Figure 10.14c).
- Left ventricular hypertrophy, systole:
  - AS – LVH – systole (Figure 10.14d).
- Anatomy with color flow Doppler across valve:
  - AS – color – AS (Figure 10.14e).
  - AS – color – AR (aortic regurgitation) (Figure 10.14f).
- Aortic valve annulus measurement:
  - AS – valve annulus (Figure 10.14g).
- Balloon position across aortic valve:
  - AS – balloon position (Figure 10.14h).
- Aortic valve post-angioplasty:
  - AS – valve – postballoon (Figure 10.14i).

SUPRAVALVAR AORTIC STENOSIS

- 2D image of anatomy:
  - SupraAS 2D (Figure 10.15a).

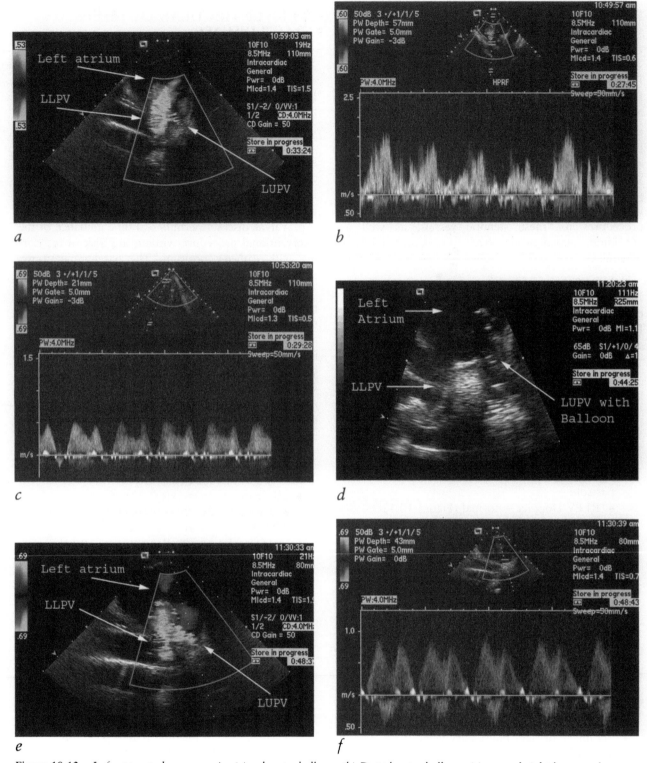

Figure 10.12 *Left upper pulmonary vein: (a) color, preballoon; (b) Doppler, preballoon; (c) normal right lower pulmonary vein Doppler, for comparison; (d) balloon; (e) color, postballoon; (f) Doppler, postballoon. LLPV = left lower pulmonary vein; LUPV = left upper pulmonary vein.*

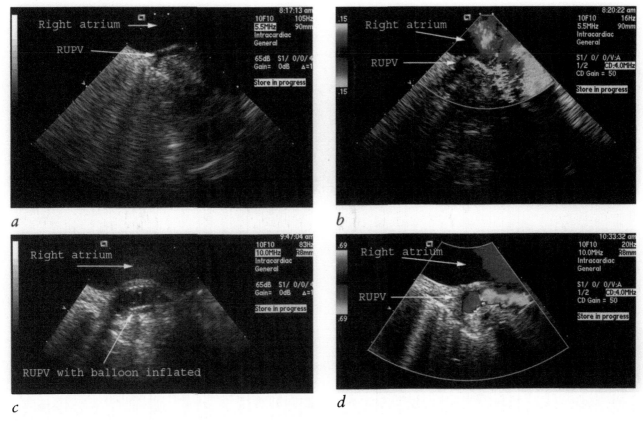

Figure 10.13 *Right upper pulmonary vein (RUPV): (a) 2D; (b) color, preballoon; (c) balloon; (d) color, postballoon.*

- Color Doppler flow:
  - SupraAS – color (Figure 10.15b).
- Spectral Doppler measurement of gradient:
  - SupraAS – Doppler (Figure 10.15c).
- Catheter position:
  - SupraAS – catheter position (Figure 10.15d).

ADULT CONGENITAL HEART DISEASE

ANATOMY

There are many potential indications for ICE in the growing field of congenital heart disease, as patients with various palliations reach adulthood. Many of these patients are exceedingly difficult to image from standard transthoracic windows, given residual lung disease and surgical scarring. Other imaging modalities must therefore be used, including transesophageal echocardiography, computed tomography (CT) angiography, and magnetic resonance imaging (MRI). However, in those patients already undergoing a cardiac catheterization or electrophysiology study under conscious sedation, ICE is a useful tool to assess palliated anatomy and function, while also improving guidance of any procedure.

TETRALOGY OF FALLOT (TOF), AS CASE EXAMPLE

- Residual VSD, 2D image:
  - TOF – VSD – 2D (Figure 10.16a).
- Residual VSD, color flow Doppler:
  - TOF – VSD – TR – color (tricuspid regurgitation) (Figure 10.16b).
- Upturned left ventricular apex due to right ventricular dilatation and hypertrophy, as seen from the right ventricle:
  - TOF – upturned apex (Figure 10.16c).

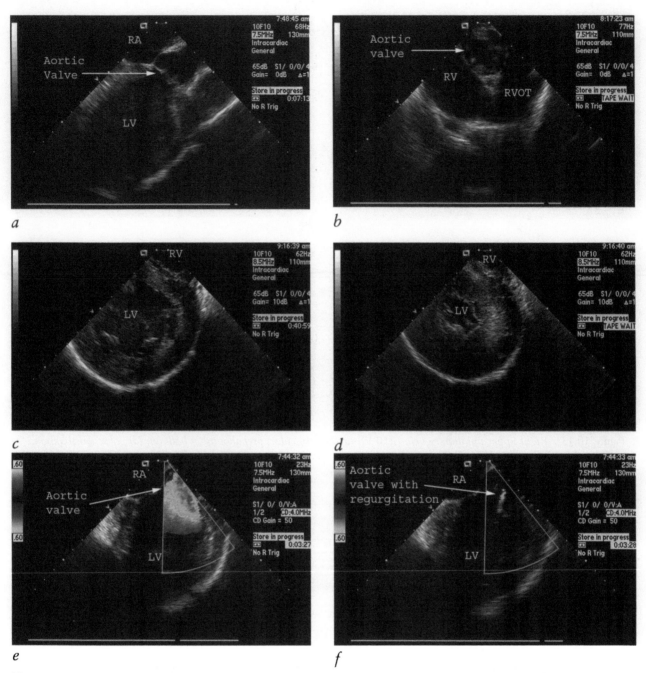

Figure 10.14 *Aortic stenosis (AS): (a) long axis (LAX) 2D; (b) valve, preballoon; (c) left ventricular hypertrophy (LVH), diastole; (d) LVH systole; (e) AS, color; (f) aortic regurgitation (AR), color; (g) valve annulus; (h) balloon position; (i) valve, postballoon. Ao = Aorta; LA = left atrium; PV = pulmonary vein; RA = right atrium; RVOT = right ventricular outflow tract.*

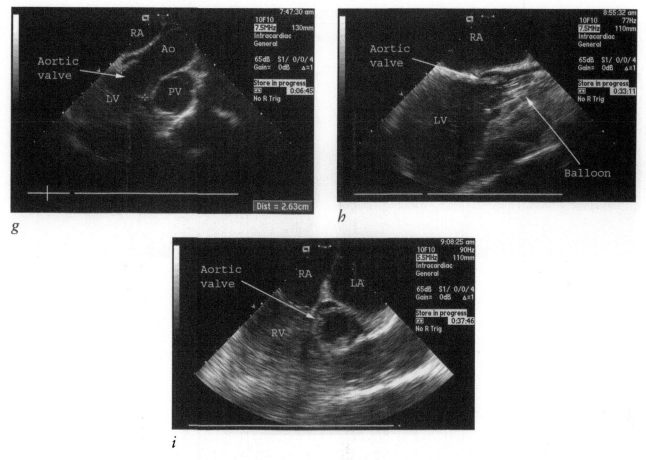

Figure 10.14 *Continued*

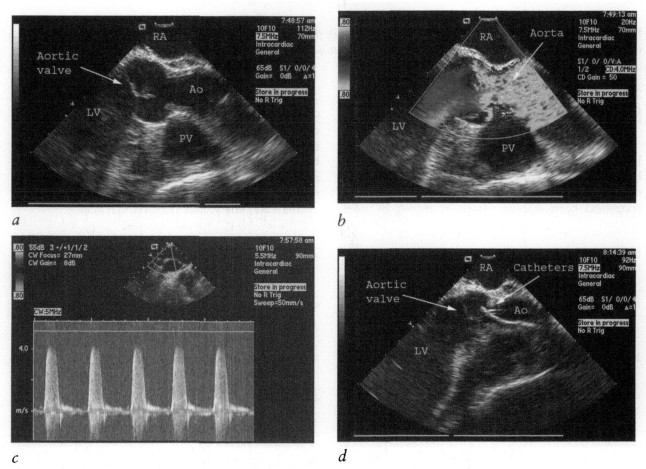

Figure 10.15 *Supravalvar aortic stenosis (SupraAS): (a) 2D; (b) color; (c) Doppler; (d) catheter position. Ao = Aorta; LA = left atrium; LV = left ventricle; PV = pulmonary vein; RA = right atrium; RV = right ventricle.*

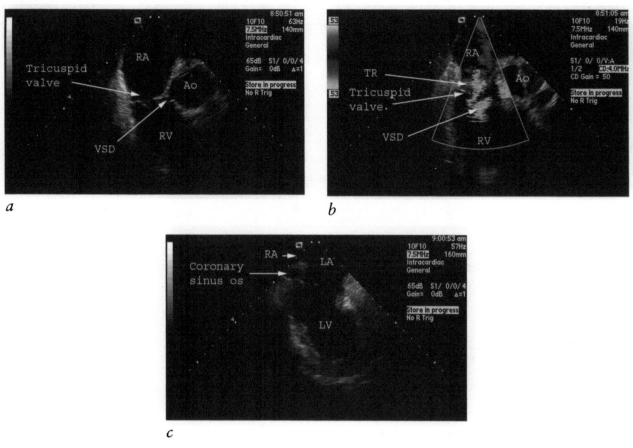

Figure 10.16   *Tetralogy of fallout (TOF): (a) residual VSD, 2D; (b) residual VSD, 2D color, with tricuspid regurgitation (TR); (c) upturned apex. Ao = Aorta; LA = left atrium; RA = right atrium; RV = right ventricle; VSD = ventricular septal defect.*

CONCLUSION

In the short time since its clinical introduction, ICE has demonstrated its utility in the management of complex arrhythmias and more simple forms of congenital heart disease. However, its use in more complex forms of congenital heart disease is still expanding, correlating with ever-expanding catheter-based interventions. This chapter should therefore be seen as a beginning of a new stage, in which multiple imaging modalities can be used simultaneously to accomplish more complex procedures with greater ease, safety, and improved outcomes.

REFERENCES

1. Packer DL, Stevens CL, Curley MG, et al. Intracardiac phased-array imaging: methods and initial clinical experience with high resolution, under blood visualization: initial experience with phased-array ultrasound. J Am Coll Cardiol 2002; 39: 509–16.

2. Bruce CJ, Nishimura RA, Rihal CS, et al. Intracardiac echocardiography in the interventional catheterization laboratory: preliminary experience with a novel, phased-array transducer. Am J Cardiol 2002; 89: 635–40.

3. Rhodes JF, Qureshi AM, Preminger TA, et al. Intracardiac echocardiography during transcatheter interventions for congenital heart disease. Am J Cardiol 2003; 92: 1482–4.

4. Arlettaz R, Archer N, Wilkinson AR. Natural history of innocent murmurs in newborn babies: controlled echocardiographic study. Arch Dis Child Fetal Neonatal Ed 1998; 78: F166–70.

5. Konstantinides S, Geibel A, Olschewski M, et al. A comparison of surgical and medical therapy for atrial septal defect in adults. N Engl J Med 1995; 333: 469–73.

6. Silversides CK, Siu SC, McLaughlin PR, et al. Symptomatic atrial arrhythmias and transcatheter closure of atrial septal defects in adult patients. Heart 2004; 90: 1194–8.

Chapter 11   Intrapericardial echocardiography: a novel catheter-based approach to cardiac imaging

Ana Clara Tude Rodrigues, Andre d'Avila, Vivek Y Reddy, and Eduardo Saad

The ability to visualize relevant cardiac structures with intracardiac echocardiography (ICE) involves placing a catheter-based ultrasound probe through the vasculature into the heart. ICE allows for precise imaging of the relationship of the mapping/ablation catheters with the cardiac anatomy, subsequently enhancing procedural efficacy and safety and reducing fluoroscopy exposure times. Fluoroscopy times are significant issues during prolonged procedures.

This chapter summarizes our initial experience with a novel catheter-based approach to cardiac imaging: the use of intrapericardial echocardiography (IPE). This non-surgical transthoracic technique involves the subxiphoid percutaneous introduction of a Tuohy needle into the pericardial space in the absence of a pericardial effusion.[1] Through this needle, a guidewire, an introducer sheath, and eventually catheters are inserted and used for epicardial mapping and ablation. Since access to the pericardial sac can be achieved with this approach, we postulated that unobstructed echocardiographic windows may allow for detailed imaging of the heart from within the pericardial space. To this end, these results (Figures 11.1–11.11) establish the experimental proof-of-principle (goats and swine) for future work in the use of this novel imaging modality during interventional cardiology procedures.[2]

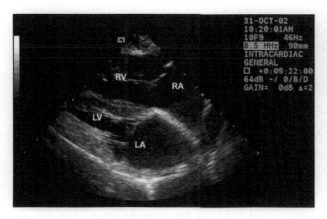

Figure 11.1 *Posterolateral positioning of the IPE probe showing a four-chamber view of the heart. RV = right ventricle; LV = left ventricle; LA = left atrium, RA = right atrium.*

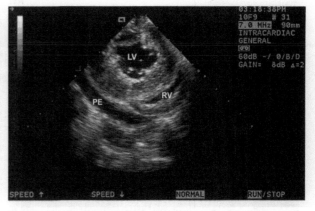

Figure 11.2 *Posterior positioning of the IPE probe displaying a short-axis view of the left ventricle at the level of papillary muscles. LV = left ventricle, RV = right ventricle; PE = pericardial effusion.*

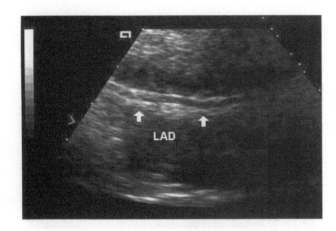

Figure 11.3 *A detailed image of the left anterior descending coronary artery (LAD) achieved by imaging the left ventricle in a modified short-axis view, focusing on the interventricular septum.*

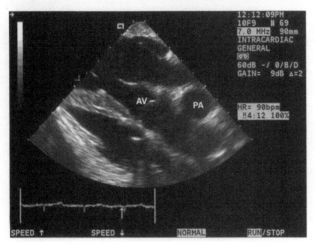

Figure 11.4 *A five-chamber view of the heart displaying the aortic valve (AV) and initial segment of the ascending aorta, obtained with the IPE probe positioned posterior to the heart. PA = pulmonary artery.*

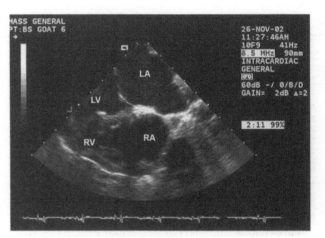

Figure 11.5 *A four-chamber view of the heart showing the interatrial septum, fossa ovalis, and the right pulmonary vein ostium. RV = right ventricle; LV = left ventricle; LA = left atrium; RA = right atrium.*

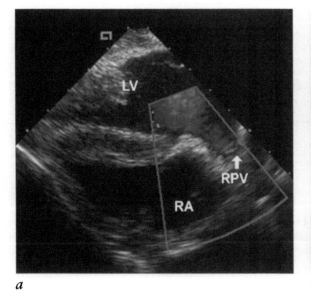

a

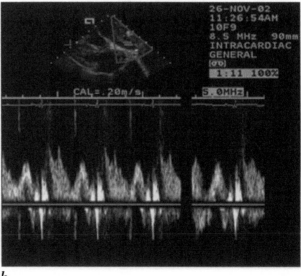

b

Figure 11.6 *Color flow mapping (a) and pulsed-wave Doppler (b) was used to demonstrate right pulmonary venous (RPV) flow. RA = right atrium; RV = right ventricle.*

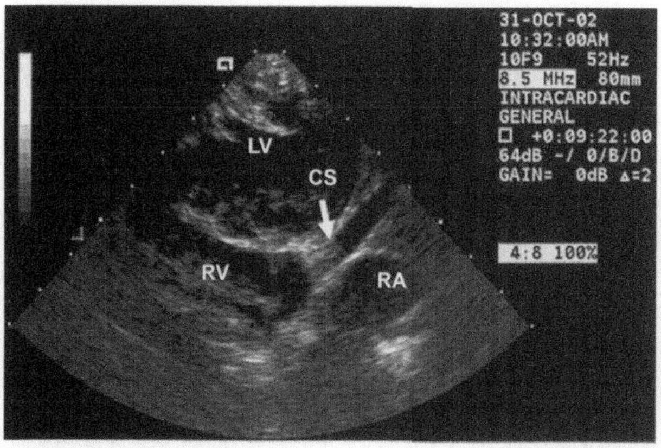

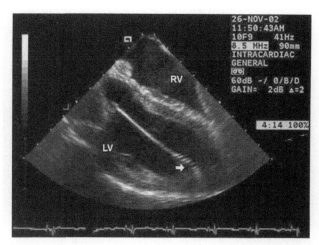

Figure 11.7 *Posterior placement of the catheter provided a longitudinal view of the coronary sinus (CS), adjacent to its entry site (arrow). RV = right ventricle; LV = left ventricle; RA = right atrium.*

Figure 11.10 *The ablation catheter can be visualized in the left ventricle. The tip of the catheter (arrow) is adjacent to the apex. RV = right ventricle; LV = left ventricle.*

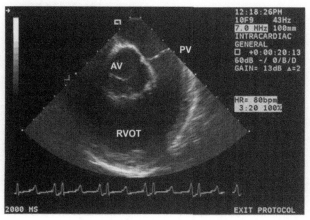

Figure 11.8 *With the IPE probe located superiorly, images of the aortic valve (AV), right ventricular outflow tract (RVOT), main pulmonary artery, and pulmonic valve (PV) are displayed.*

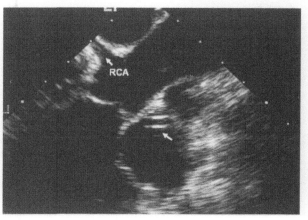

Figure 11.11 *Ablation catheter (arrow) visualized in the left atrium. Aortic valve and right coronary artery (RCA) are also seen.*

ACKNOWLEDGMENT

Figures 11.1–11.11 are reprinted from Reference 2 with permission from the American Society of Echocardiography.

REFERENCES

1. Sosa E, Scanavacca M, d'Avila A, Pilleggi F. A new technique to perform epicardial mapping in the electrophysiology laboratory. J Cardiovasc Electrophysiol 1996; 7: 531–6.
2. Rodrigues AC, d'Avila A, Houghtaling C, Rushmi JN, Picard M, Reddy VY. Intrapericardial echocardiography: a novel catheter-based approach to cardiac imaging. J Am Soc Echocardiogr 2004; 3: 269–74.

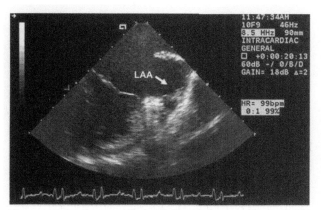

Figure 11.9 *Image of the left atrial appendage (LAA) with posterior intrapericardial echocardiography catheter placement.*

Chapter 12   Three-dimensional echocardiography – future applications in interventional cardiology

Hsuan-Hung Chuang, Tamas Szili-Torok, Luc J Jordaens, and Takahiro Shiota

INTRODUCTION

Three-dimensional (3D) echocardiographic imaging has been introduced as a tool to improve the assessment of both morphologic and functional parameters of the cardiovascular system. With the technologic advances, it is now a clinical reality and a practical tool for performing 3D echocardiography using transthoracic or transesophageal acoustic windows, in both adults and children. As regards its potential, most excitement lies in its ability to evaluate a specific region of interest in any desired orientation and to capture accurate quantitative data without using any geometric assumption, as in two-dimensional (2D) echocardiography. Real-time (RT) 3D echocardiography with matrix-array transducers is the most promising approach, but there are still some limitations. As we move towards more catheter-based therapies in this new millennium, 3D echocardiography will play a complementary role in providing the precise dynamic information on cardiac structure and function. We will review the clinical applications of 3D echocardiography in the current realm of interventional cardiology.

THREE-DIMENSIONAL ECHOCARDIOGRAPHY

Compared to other state-of-the-art developments in the realm of cardiovascular imaging, such as computed tomography (CT) imaging and magnetic resonance imaging (MRI), the evolution of 3D echocardiography has been slow, despite its appearance on the scene in the early 1970s, and the subsequent demonstration of the superiority of 3D echocardiography in the determination of ventricular volume, ventricular mass, or valvular orifice area in the late 1990s. With technologic advances, the slow laborious methods of image acquisition have given way to a faster acquisition system, based on either mechanical rotation of a phased-array transducer or on electronic beam steering with mosaic transducers. Of the three common methods of acquisition of temporal and positional image data – i.e. positional locators, rotational systems, and RT volumetric scanning – RT 3D echocardiography with matrix-array transducers is the most promising technique as it avoids the need for respiratory gating to reduce spatial motion artifacts, as well as the need for offline post-processing of data. The incorporation of this technology into transesophageal or intracardiac echocardiography probes will undoubtedly open the way for its increasing use in interventional cardiology.[1,2]

CLINICAL APPLICATIONS

ASSESSMENT OF CHAMBER VOLUME AND FUNCTION

Accurate assessment of left ventricular (LV) volume, ejection fraction, and segmental wall motion abnormalities is important in clinical decision-making. Echocardiography is the imaging modality that is most commonly applied in practice to derive the ejection fraction. The application of biplane Simpson's rule in 2D echocardiography has considerably improved the accuracy of LV volume measurements, especially in both symmetric and asymmetric left ventricles. Software-based algorithms for automatic endocardial border detection and online

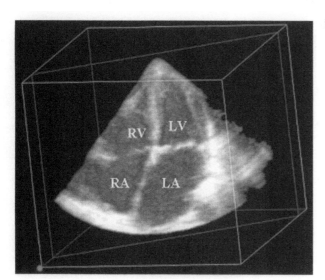

Figure 12.1 *Three-dimensional presentation of an anatomically correct apical four-chamber view.*

calculation of LV volume and ejection fraction have also been utilized. However, the assumptions about LV geometry remain a limitation of conventional 2D echocardiography. It has been shown that 3D echocardiography provides an accurate and reproducible method for LV quantification, mainly by avoiding the use of geometric assumptions, as in 2D echocardiography.[3]

The multidirectional beam-steering capability of the newer live 3D echocardiography enables visualization of two views of the heart simultaneously, and is useful for assessment of ejection fraction in dilated cardiomyopathy (Figure 12.1). There have been numerous studies[4–10] comparing quantification of LV volume and function by 3D echocardiography with MRI, and a good correlation has been observed. Some studies showed that end-systolic volume and end-diastolic volume tend to be underestimated on 3D echocardiography studies. With further advances in technologies, contrast enhancement, improvement in spatial resolution, and development of new 3D echocardiography automated endocardial border detection, 3D echocardiography has great potential to become an important technique for volume and function assessment.

ASSESSMENT OF REGIONAL WALL MOTION ABNORMALITIES, MYOCARDIAL PERFUSION, AND LEFT VENTRICULAR DYSSYNCHRONY

McPherson et al[11] used 3D echocardiography to study the effect of acute ischemia on diastolic function in dogs in 1987. Subsequently, other studies showed

that quantification of the extent of regional wall motion abnormalities by 3D echocardiography provides a better and more accurate estimate of the infarct size than can be obtained with 2D echocardiography. However, it remains to be proven that patient outcomes would be altered by a more accurate echocardiographic estimation of infarct size.[6,12] This new echocardiographic technique may prove useful in further experimental studies of infarct-modifying therapies, including stem cell injection, and in the assessment of LV regional changes in various disease states (Figure 12.2).

We also know that neither the extent of patency nor the severity of stenosis of the infarct-related artery indicate the extent of microvascular integrity. Assessment of regional myocardial perfusion may be possible in combination with myocardial contrast agents. This can be delineated by manually injecting agitated bubbles either into the LV cavity or directly into the coronary arteries, and subsequently observing their transit through the complete coronary vasculature. Areas that do not fill with contrast are "at risk" for myocardial necrosis. Chen and colleagues[13] studied the spatial distribution of myocardial perfusion defects using RT 3D echocardiography combined with myocardial contrast echocardiography (MCE) (Figure 12.3). In-vitro myocardial mass was used as the control to validate the feasibility and accuracy in determining perfusion defects. It was demonstrated that, following coronary artery occlusion, MCE combined with 3D echocardiography showed a high correlation with the measurement of underperfused myocardial mass and percentage of total LV mass by in-vitro assessment.

The use of 3D echocardiography has allowed a better spatial appreciation of the architecture of a coronary artery or its territory. These findings have important clinical significance, as the size of the underperfused myocardium is an important predictor of cardiac function and prognosis. Other studies[14–16] have confirmed the feasibility and accuracy of dynamic 3D echocardiography in the determination of wall motion abnormalities, and also shown that estimation of the myocardial mass of perfusion defects by dynamic 3D echocardiography closely correlates with those defined by nuclear scintigraphy and triphenyltetrazolium staining. A strong correlation was also observed between dynamic 3D echocardiography and MRI (a reference standard for infarcted tissue detection) in the measurement of underperfused myocardial mass. A potential application is to use 3D echocardiographic reconstruction to assist in radiofrequency ablation treatment for post-infarct ventricular arrhythmia, as one can visualize the aneurysmal, dyskinetic, or dysplastic segments, thereby

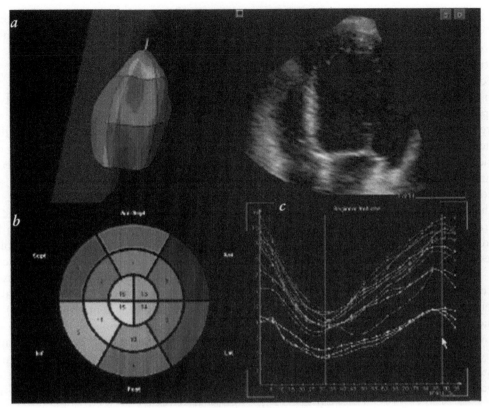

Figure 12.2 *A three-dimensional left ventricular regional wall motion and volumetric analysis. (a) Spatial display of the left ventricle; ventricular regions are color coded. (b) Regional volumes are displayed as a "bull's eye". (c) Changes in regional volumes over the cardiac cycle are automatically calculated and displayed.*

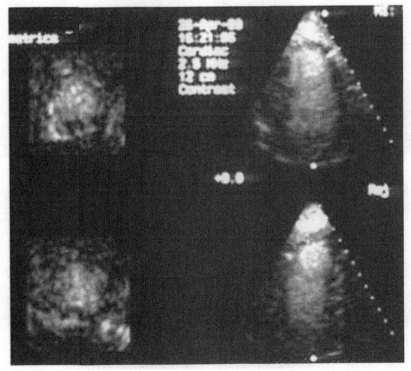

Figure 12.3 *A three-dimensional echocardiography with contrast. Four different two-dimensional cut planes (four- and two-chamber apical views and base and mid short-axis views) could be simultaneously visualized during contrast injection.*

avoiding complications. In brief, 3D echocardiography has shown great promise in its ability to rapidly acquire and visualize data, which facilitates rapid evaluation of acute myocardial infarction, estimation of cardiac function and of LV remodeling, and prediction of survival rates in clinical settings.[12–17]

Tissue Doppler imaging (TDI) is the imaging modality currently used to assess the most delayed ventricular site before implantation of a resynchronization device. Dynamic 3D echocardiography combined with automated contour analysis has been found to be feasible to determine mechanical asynchrony during LV contraction and the most delayed contraction site of the left ventricle. In a clinical study by Krenning et al, 3D echocardiographic images were obtained during resynchronization device implantation.[18] They showed that simultaneous electrical stimulation of both ventricles with biventricular pacing in patients with interventricular conduction disturbance and advanced heart failure improved hemodynamics and resulted in increased exercise tolerance and quality of life. The results suggested that fast reconstruction of the LV from 3D echocardiography is feasible for the selection of the optimal pacing site, and therefore valuable in evaluation and guiding resynchronization device implantation.

ASSESSMENT OF CARDIAC VALVES

Surgery is often required for patients with advanced valvular heart disease. Three-dimensional echocardiographic imaging is able to provide excellent "surgical views", prior to opening the heart, with great detail and precision (Figure 12.4). First, the degree of stenosis (valve area) and morphologic and functional alterations in regurgitant valves can be assessed quantitatively. When combined with 3D-color Doppler data, the visualization of flows in 3D could allow a better qualitative and quantitative assessment of their size and severity; it has the potential to display the flow convergence zone (Figure 12.5) and quantify the regurgitant volume. It is also capable of distinguishing particular destructive substructures of the valves and the valvular apparatus. This is especially important in the management of patients with infective endocarditis, as it can aid in deciding

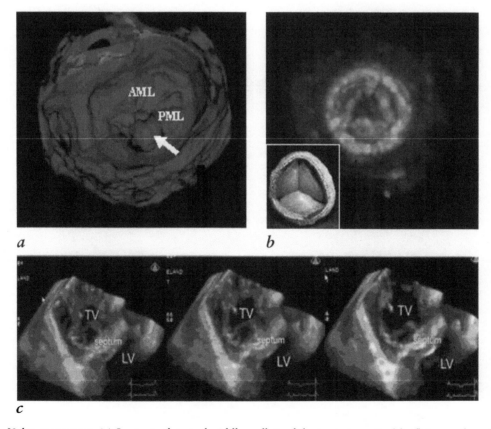

Figure 12.4   *Valve assessment. (a) Severe prolapse of middle scallop of the posterior mitral leaflet, seen from the left atrium (surgical view). (b) Enface views of the Carpentier–Edwards tissue valve at the mitral position. (c) Enface view of native tricuspid valve at three different times during a cardiac cycle.*

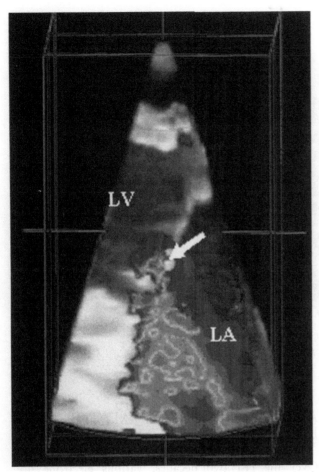

Figure 12.5 *Flow convergence (arrow) towards the mitral regurgitant orifice in a patient with mitral regurgitation.*

when and how to intervene. Lastly, percutaneous valve repair/reconstruction and valvuloplasty can also be facilitated through 3D echocardiography.

Prognosis of coronary artery disease depends on a multitude of factors, including the degree of LV dysfunction, presence of inducible ischemia, viable dysfunctioning myocardium, degree of coronary artery lesions, and so forth. Mitral regurgitation (MR) is an independent predictor of cardiovascular mortality, and results from many factors, such as papillary muscle dysfunction, mitral annular dilatation, LV remodeling, and degree of viability. In fact, "ischemic" MR has been the subject of much interest to cardiologists, echocardiographers, cardiothoracic surgeons, and most recently interventional cardiologists. Advances in 3D echocardiography have allowed us to address the mechanism and optimal treatment of these MRs.[19–21] Otsuji et al[19] showed that the development of MR relates strongly to changes in the 3D geometry of the mitral apparatus, with implications for approaches to restore a more favorable configuration. In practical terms, it is suggested that surgical approaches could benefit patients by restoring

overall mitral valve geometry towards normal. In dilated cardiomyopathy, correction of significant MR improves patient's symptoms and eventually leads to a better outcome.[22] Surgical correction of substantial MR is often considered during revascularization surgery. At present, there are two experimental percutaneous approaches to correction of MR: edge-to-edge mitral valve repair technique and catheter-based annuloplasty through the coronary sinus. The edge-to-edge technique mimics the Alfieri procedure by securing the two leaflets together at the site of maximal regurgitation, thereby creating a "double-orifice" mitral valve (Figure 12.6). This is performed through transcatheter delivery of a clip (Evalve, Inc., Redwood City, CA). Retraction of the device with the clip in the open position allows the free leaflet edge to be grasped in systole at the time of closure. The clip is closed after confirmation of optimal site of device deployment with satisfactory hemodynamics. Real-time 3D echocardiography with transesophageal echocardiography would allow a better appreciation of the valve anatomy and reduce the fluoroscopic time. The other interventional method entails the insertion of a constraint device through the coronary sinus. Precise visualization of the opening of the coronary sinus and relevant anatomy is definitely needed before the procedure is contemplated. Three-dimensional echocardiography and/or CT scan reconstruction of the working anatomy would definitely be helpful.

Prolapse of the mitral valve is another frequently encountered problem in clinical cardiology. Over the years, transesophageal 2D echocardiography has provided important information, with regard to structure, morphology, and function, that has guided management. But, it was using 3D echocardiography that the mitral annulus was found to have a saddle-like shape, with the high point of the saddle (i.e. closest to left atrium) positioned in an anterior–posterior axis and the low points (i.e. closer to apex) in the medial–lateral axis.[23] One can identify the exact segment or scallop of the leaflet that is pathologic (Figure 12.7). In mitral stenosis, volume-rendered 3D echocardiography can be used to measure the exact orifice area of the mitral valve and identify the morphologic abnormalities that may predict the success or failure of valvuloplasty, such as pliability and thickening of leaflets, degree of commissural fusion, and extent of calcification. From the 3D data-set, the short-axis section that intersects the tip of the mitral valve leaflets on the smallest orifice is identified and the area of stenosis is obtained thereafter by planimetry. This circumvents the inaccuracies of the 2D echocardiographic assessment due to beam malalignment and difficulty in locating the tip precisely. The accuracy of this method of assessment

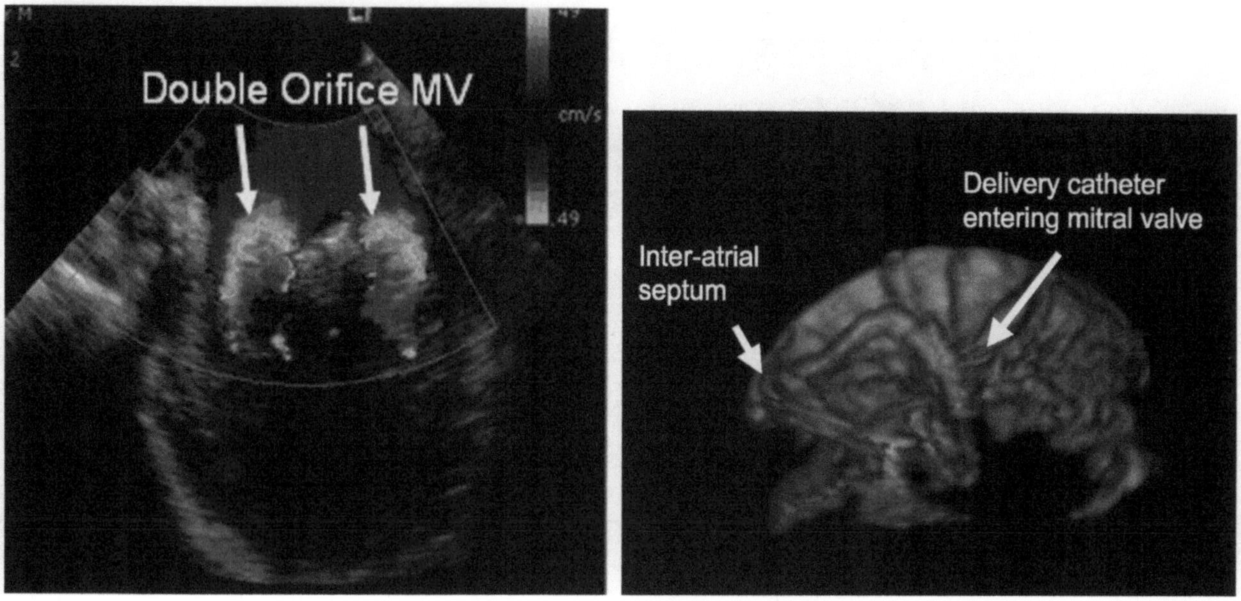

a   *b*

Figure 12.6 *(a) This patient with severe mitral regurgitation that underwent percutaneous edge-to-edge repair of the mitral valve, creating a double-orifice mitral valve with forward flow seen through the double orifices. (b) Delivery catheter in the left atrium seen passing through the mitral valve.*

was confirmed in clinical studies that showed an excellent correlation with actual mitral valve area (MVA) found at surgery.

In addition, RT 3D echocardiography has shown its superiority in evaluating the MVA in the immediate post-valvuloplasty period. Directly following a percutaneous mitral valvuloplasty, the pressure half-time method has been shown to have a poor agreement with invasive data. Numerous reasons account for this inaccuracy, including the development of an atrial septal defect (ASD) in many patients after the valvuloplasty, and the fact that the pressure half-time method assumes that left atrial and LV compliances remain stable. As such, this assumption made in the pressure half-time method is not valid immediately post-valvuloplasty because rapid changes in the left atrial pressure and LV filling occur in this setting, affecting the compliance of both the left atrium and ventricle. The RT 3D echocardiographic MVA assessment better agrees with the invasively derived MVA before and in the immediate post-valvuloplasty period. Likewise, using paraplane and anyplane sections, the morphology, severity, and exact orifice area of aortic stenosis and other valvular disease can be ascertained. In infective endocarditis, 3D echocardiography can provide more information on the presence and degree of structural involvement, and on the extension of damage, as 3D echocardiography is able to provide the enface views of the valve and any perforation.[24]

ASSESSMENT OF ANATOMY FOR ELECTROPHYSIOLOGY STUDIES

Over the last two decades, various electrophysiologic mapping and transcatheter radiofrequency ablation techniques have been established as one of the treatment options for many cardiac tachyarrhythmias; the success rates in most reported series are high, but in some cases are still suboptimal. The failure to achieve the desired outcome is in part due to mistargeted lesion creation or ablation. Since the arrhythmia substrate is frequently associated with certain anatomic structures or morphologic variants, improved imaging has an increasing role in the improvement of these treatments. Classical imaging techniques may be unable to visualize structures involved in arrhythmia mechanisms and therapy. For example, valves can exist at the os of the coronary sinus, which can serve as an obstacle for diagnostic and pacing catheters. Linear structures such as the tendon of Todaro, the ligament of Marshall, and the crista terminalis may be identified (Figure 12.7).[25] In addition, 3D reconstruction using ICE has also been studied to guide the selection of optimal interatrial septum pacing sites in the management of paroxysmal atrial fibrillation (Figures 12.8 and 12.9). Intracardiac echocardiography has been utilized to visualize the left ventricular outflow tract (LVOT) by either positioning the catheter close to the anterior interatrial septum (His bundle region),

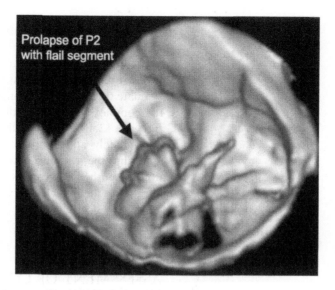

Figure 12.7 *Prolapse of P2 (arrow) segment with frail segment seen in real-time 3D transesophageal echocardiography.*

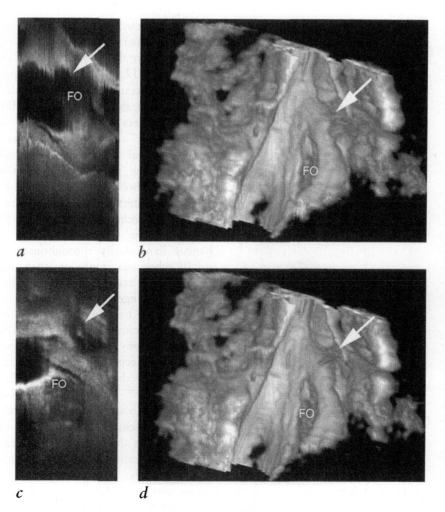

Figure 12.8 *a–d Three-dimensional image of atrial lead (arrow) in front of the anterior–superior edge of the muscular interatrial septum and the membrane of fossa ovalis (FO). Reproduced with permission from Szili-Torok T et al, Interatrial septum pacing guided by three-dimensional intracardiac echocardiography. J Am Coll Cardiol 2002; 40: 2139–43.*

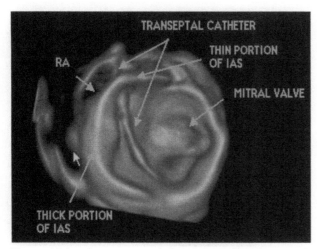

Figure 12.9 *Orientation of the transeptal catheter with relation to the interatrial septum.*

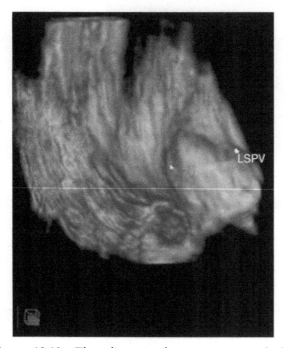

Figure 12.10 *Three-dimensional reconstruction of the pulmonary vein region with intracardiac echocardiography. LSPV = Left superior pulmonary vein.*

or at the base of right ventricular outflow tract, whereby the ostium of the left main coronary artery can be visualized. In ventricular tachycardia originating near the LVOT, 3D reconstruction can

possibly guide catheter ablation by permitting the identification of anatomic landmarks, including the aortic root, endocardial contact, and ablation electrode. Preliminary studies have been conducted to evaluate the use of 3D reconstruction in understanding the complex anatomy of the pulmonary vein ostium (Figure 12.10). The utility of 3D imaging will undoubtedly add another dimension to guiding and assessing the completeness of radiofrequency ablation and other electrophysiologic procedures, and to improving the overall safety.

ASSESSMENT OF CONGENITAL HEART DISEASE

The ability of 3D echocardiography to evaluate a specific region of interest in any desired orientation is of particular importance in the assessment of the various defects and severity of congenital heart disease.[26–28] Atrial septal defect and patent foramen ovale (PFO) are the most common cardiac abnormalities (Figure 12.11). They predispose to cerebral ischemia as a result of paradoxical thromboembolism by right-to-left shunting under conditions or physiologic maneuvers that raise right atrial pressure. As discussed above, transcatheter occlusion of these interatrial communications has shown great promise in the primary and secondary prevention of thromboembolic strokes. The results are comparable to surgical intervention. In patients with complex defects, 2D echocardiography may underestimate the size of the defect. In addition, the ASD area changes dynamically throughout the cardiac cycle, and 2D echocardiography or other imaging techniques have failed to recognize this diastolic–systolic difference. The changes in the defect areas are not only parallel to the heart axis from base to apex but are also perpendicular to the axis. Three-dimensional echocardiography allows enface views of the atrial septum and accurate measurement of the maximal diameter and the systolic and diastolic areas of the defects.[29,30] The information obtained enables the operator to decide on how these defects should be closed or select the appropriate size and type of device. During the procedure, 3D echocardiography allows visualization and optimal deployment of the closure devices, and assessment of periprocedural complications.

In recent years, transcatheter devices have also been used to close ventricular septal defects (VSDs).

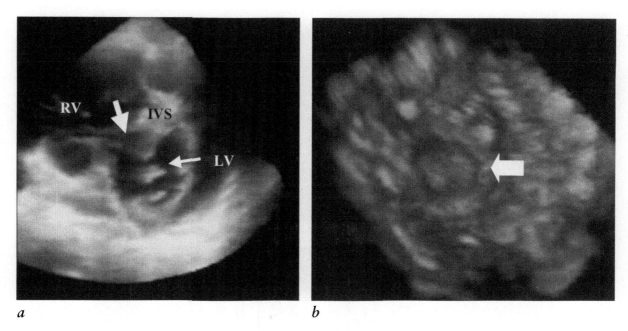

a　　　　　　　　　　　　　　　　　*b*

Figure 12.11 *(a) Sagittal view of a large muscular interventricular defect (large arrow), with irregular borders. (b) Enface view of an atrial septal defect (arrow), seen from the right atrium in a 7-year-old girl.*

Various devices have been used with variable success, including the Rashkind double-umbrella device, the Bard clamshell device, the Sideris button device, and Gianturco coil. The advantages of the percutaneous closure technique include the avoidance of morbidity related to thoracotomy and cardiopulmonary bypass, and the reduced hospitalization. Early results of transcatheter closure using a variety of devices have reported few complications.[26,31–33] Nonetheless, the interventional cardiologist should be aware of the relationship of the VSD to the adjacent structures.[34] For example, the inlet portion of the ventricular septum from the right ventricular view is obscured by the septal leaflet of the tricuspid valve, whereas the corresponding part on the left side is the LVOT. One important structural consideration is the atrioventricular conduction bundle, which lies in close proximity to the posterior–inferior border of the perimembranous VSD, and in the superior margin of a muscular VSD; another is the proximity of the VSD to the arterial valves and the atrioventricular valves. Patients are thus carefully selected by strict criteria. Clinical series have suggested that most morphologic forms of perimembranous defects that are not complicated by septal malalignment or valvular prolapse can be potentially amenable to device closure after careful assessment of size, shape, and distance from crucial structures. Three-dimensional echocardiography will undoubtedly provide better visualization of such structures from all angles.

POTENTIAL UTILITIES IN OTHER INTERVENTIONAL PROCEDURES IN CARDIOLOGY

Alcohol septal ablation in hypertrophic cardiomyopathy

We have previously reported the use of RT 3D echocardiography in planning for septal myectomy in a young man with asymmetrical hypertrophic cardiomyopathy with severe LVOT obstruction[35] (Figure 12.12). A good spatial assessment of the LVOT, the extent of maximal septal thickness, and the extent of systolic mitral leaflet-to-septal contact are all important factors that help the surgeons decide the site and size of the septal myectomy. In addition, the technique can also be used for monitoring complications post-myectomy, such as septal perforator coronary artery–left ventricle fistula.[36]

Cardiac masses

Three-dimensional echocardiography has the ability to provide 2D cut-plane displays from any chosen location and direction within the 3D datasets. This information on the appearance, the location, and the extension of any intracardiac mass helps to determine the likelihood of pathology and the subsequent management strategies.[37,38] Based on in-vitro validation, masses such as myxomas and

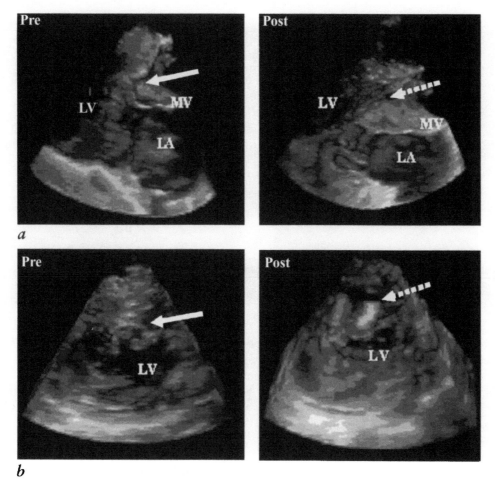

Figure 12.12   *Three-dimensional images obtained pre- and post-septal myectomy. (a) Parasternal long-axis and (b) short-axis images demonstrating the marked systolic anterior motion of the mitral valve pre-surgery (full arrow) with left ventricular outflow tract (LVOT) obstruction. The (LVOT) is widely patent post-myectomy (broken arrows).*

vegetations have been quantitatively assessed and their volume and size derived. In this way, 3D imaging again provides a better assessment of the dimensions of these masses. By viewing the masses from multiple positions within the 3D datasets, one can avoid the artifactual measurements sometimes obtained with 2D imaging.

CONCLUSION

With future advances in digital imaging processing hardware and software, the integration of 3D echocardiography into conventional scanner and operator-friendly applications will reduce the time and effort required for 3D-image acquisition, reconstruction, and quantitative analysis. Combination with color Doppler data may lead to more precise quantitation of valve stenosis and regurgitation. The advent of real-time 3D imaging and color Doppler will generate 3D images directly on the screen during evaluation. The incorporation of other echocardiographic modalities such as tissue Doppler imaging and contrast echocardiography into the 3D-display format could further enhance our perception of cardiac structure and function. At present, the additional information in intervention or surgical decision-making can be addressed and therefore justify the use of this evolving technology in clinical practice.[39]

REFERENCES

1. Sheikh K, Smith SW, von Ramm O, Kisslo J. Real-time, three-dimensional echocardiography: feasibility and initial use. Echocardiography 1991; 8: 119–25.
2. De Castro S, Yao J, Pandian NG. Three-dimensional echocardiography: clinical relevance and application. Am J Cardiol 1998; 81: 96–102G.
3. Esh-Broder E, Ushakov FB, Imbar T, Yagel S. Application of freehand three-dimensional echocardiography in the evaluation of fetal cardiac ejection fraction: a preliminary study. Ultrasound Obstet Gynecol 2004; 23: 546–51.
4. Krenning BJ, Voormolen MM, Roelandt JR. Assessment of left ventricular function by three-dimensional echocardiography. Cardiovasc Ultrasound 2003; 1: 12.
5. Buck T, Hunold P, Wentz KU, et al. Tomographic three-dimensional echocardiographic determination of chamber size and systolic function in patients with left ventricular aneurysm: comparison to magnetic resonance imaging, cineventriculography, and two-dimensional echocardiography. Circulation 1997; 96: 4286–97.
6. Gopal AS, Keller AM, Rigling R, et al. Left ventricular volume and endocardial surface area by three-dimensional echocardiography: comparison with two-dimensional echocardiography and nuclear magnetic resonance imaging in normal subjects. J Am Coll Cardiol 1993; 22: 258–70.
7. Gopal AS, Keller AM, Shen Z, et al. Three-dimensional echocardiography: in vitro and in vivo validation of left ventricular mass and comparison with conventional echocardiographic methods. J Am Coll Cardiol 1994; 24: 504–13.
8. Gopal AS, Shen Z, Sapin PM, et al. Assessment of cardiac function by three-dimensional echocardiography compared with conventional noninvasive methods. Circulation 1995; 92: 842–53.
9. Kim WY, Sogaard P, Kristensen BO, Egeblad H. Measurement of left ventricular volumes by 3-dimensional echocardiography with tissue harmonic imaging: a comparison with magnetic resonance imaging. J Am Soc Echocardiogr 2001; 14: 169–79.
10. King DL, Gopal AS, Keller AM, et al. Three-dimensional echocardiography. Advances for measurement of ventricular volume and mass. Hypertension 1994; 23: I172–9.
11. McPherson DD, Skorton DJ, Kodiyalam S, et al. Finite element analysis of myocardial diastolic function using three-dimensional echocardiographic reconstructions: application of a new method for study of acute ischemia in dogs. Circ Res 1987; 60: 674–82.
12. Sapin PM, Clarke GB, Gopal AS, et al. Validation of three-dimensional echocardiography for quantifying the extent of dyssynergy in canine acute myocardial infarction: comparison with two-dimensional echocardiography. J Am Coll Cardiol 1996; 27: 1761–70.
13. Chen LX, Wang XF, Nanda NC, et al. Real-time three-dimensional myocardial contrast echocardiography in assessment of myocardial perfusion defects. Chin Med J (Engl) 2004; 117: 337–41.
14. Yao J, De Castro S, Delabays A, et al. Bulls-eye display and quantitation of myocardial perfusion defects using three-dimensional contrast echocardiography. Echocardiography 2001; 18: 581–8.
15. De Castro S, Yao J, Fedele F, Pandian NG. Three-dimensional echocardiography in ischemic heart disease. Coron Artery Dis 1998; 9: 427–34.
16. De Castro S, Yao J, Magni G, et al. Three-dimensional echocardiographic assessment of the extension of dysfunctional mass in patients with coronary artery disease. Am J Cardiol 1998; 81: 103–6G.
17. Braunwald E. Myocardial reperfusion, limitation of infarct size, reduction of left ventricular dysfunction, and improved survival. Should the paradigm be expanded? Circulation 1989; 79: 441–4.
18. Krenning BJ, Szili-Torok T, Voormolen MM, et al. Guiding and optimization of resynchronization therapy with dynamic three-dimensional echocardiography and segmental volume–time curves: a feasibility study. Eur J Heart Fail 2004; 6: 619–25.
19. Otsuji Y, Handschumacher MD, Liel-Cohen N, et al. Mechanism of ischemic mitral regurgitation with segmental left ventricular dysfunction: three-dimensional echocardiographic studies in models of acute and chronic progressive regurgitation. J Am Coll Cardiol 2001; 37: 641–8.
20. Salustri A, Becker AE, van Herwerden L, et al. Three-dimensional echocardiography of normal and pathologic mitral valve: a comparison with two-dimensional transesophageal echocardiography. J Am Coll Cardiol 1996; 27: 1502–10.
21. Levine RA, Handschumacher MD, Sanfilippo AJ, et al. Three-dimensional echocardiographic reconstruction of the mitral valve, with implications for the diagnosis of mitral valve prolapse. Circulation 1989; 80: 589–98.
22. Gatti G, Cardu G, Pugliese P. Mitral valve surgery for mitral regurgitation in patients with advanced dilated cardiomyopathy. Ital Heart J 2003; 4: 29–34.
23. Levine RA, Triulzi MO, Harrigan P, Weyman AE. The relationship of mitral annular shape to the diagnosis of mitral valve prolapse. Circulation 1987; 75: 756–67.
24. Marx GR, Sherwood MC. Three-dimensional echocardiography in congenital heart disease: a continuum of unfulfilled promises? No. A presently clinically applicable technology with an important future? Yes. Pediatr Cardiol 2002; 23: 266–85.
25. Szili-Torok T, McFadden E, Jordaens L, Roelandt J. Visualization of elusive structures using intracardiac echocardiography: insights from electrophysiology. Cardiovasc Ultrasound 2004; 2: 6.
26. Vogel M, Losch S. Dynamic three-dimensional echocardiography with a computed tomography imaging probe: initial clinical experience with transthoracic application in infants and children with congenital heart defects. Br Heart J 1994; 71: 462–7.
27. Fulton DR, Marx GR, Pandian NG, et al. Dynamic three-dimensional echocardiographic imaging of congenital heart defects in infants and children by computer-controlled tomographic parallel slicing using a single integrated ultrasound instrument. Echocardiography 1994; 11: 155–64.
28. Salustri A, Spitaels S, McGhie J, et al. Transthoracic three-dimensional echocardiography in adult patients with congenital heart disease. J Am Coll Cardiol 1995; 26: 759–67.
29. Marx GR, Fulton DR, Pandian NG, et al. Delineation of site, relative size and dynamic geometry of atrial septal defects by

real-time three-dimensional echocardiography. J Am Coll Cardiol 1995; 25: 482–90.

30. Belohlavek M, Foley DA, Gerber TC, et al. Three-dimensional ultrasound imaging of the atrial septum: normal and pathologic anatomy. J Am Coll Cardiol 1993; 22: 1673–8.

31. Lock JE, Block PC, McKay RG, et al. Transcatheter closure of ventricular septal defects. Circulation 1988; 78: 361–8.

32. Rigby ML, Redington AN. Primary transcatheter umbrella closure of perimembranous ventricular septal defect. Br Heart J 1994; 72: 368–71.

33. Kalra GS, Verma PK, Dhall A, et al. Transcatheter device closure of ventricular septal defects: immediate results and intermediate-term follow-up. Am Heart J 1999; 138: 339–44.

34. Ho SY, McCarthy KP, Rigby ML. Morphology of perimembranous ventricular septal defects: implications for transcatheter device closure. J Interv Cardiol 2004; 17: 99–108.

35. Nash PJ, Agler DA, Shin JH, et al. Images in cardiovascular medicine. Epicardial real-time 3-dimensional echocardiography during septal myectomy for obstructive hypertrophic cardiomyopathy. Circulation 2003; 108: e54–5.

36. Patel V, Nanda NC, Vengala S, et al. Live three-dimensional transthoracic echocardiographic demonstration of septal perforator coronary artery–left ventricle fistulas following myectomy. Echocardiography 2005; 22: 273–5.

37. Kupferwasser I, Mohr-Kahaly S, Erbel R, et al. Three-dimensional imaging of cardiac mass lesions by transesophageal echocardiographic computed tomography. J Am Soc Echocardiogr 1994; 7: 561–70.

38. Schwartz SL, Cao QL, Azevedo J, Pandian NG. Simulation of intraoperative visualization of cardiac structures and study of dynamic surgical anatomy with real-time three-dimensional echocardiography. Am J Cardiol 1994; 73: 501–7.

39. Abraham TP, Warner JG Jr, Kon ND, et al. Feasibility, accuracy, and incremental value of intraoperative three-dimensional transesophageal echocardiography in valve surgery. Am J Cardiol 1997; 80: 1577–82.

Chapter 13   The future of image-guided therapies in interventional electrophysiology

Dimpi Patel, Marcoen F Scholten, Robert Savage, and Vivek Reddy

INTRODUCTION

At the end of World War II, ultrasound imaging technology became critical to non-government scientists. Since then, ultrasound has played a critical role in the assessment of anatomic structures. Intracardiac echocardiography (ICE) has revolutionized intracardiac imaging in interventional electrophysiology by increasing the ability to accurately target sites, reducing fluoroscopy times, and providing the ability to immediately assess for certain complications. The implementation of ICE has effectively addressed several technical hurdles in interventional electrophysiology and has subsequently helped pave the way for other navigation imaging modalities and for further therapeutic advancements.

THE BALLOON PARADIGM

A number of "one-size-fits-all" ablation devices are being developed to rapidly, effectively, and safely isolate the pulmonary veins (PVs) to treat atrial fibrillation (AF) (Figure 13.1). Cryoballoons, laser balloons, and focused ultrasound balloons are all being experimentally employed to isolate the pulmonary veins. The cryoballoon catheter is able to create cryolesions by delivering liquid N_2O into a semicompliant balloon (18–22 mm diameter). Cryothermy is attractive for use in AF ablation because of its favorable safety profile, but the "heat load" associated with the PV blood flow makes traditional catheter designs less effective. A balloon cryoablation catheter placed at the PV ostia may

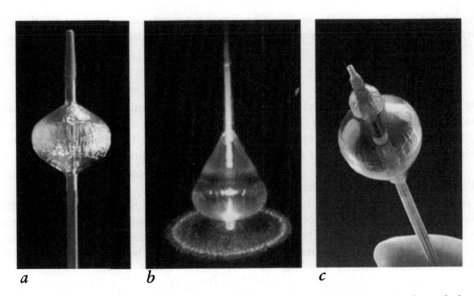

a   *b*   *c*

Figure 13.1   *(a) Cryoablation balloon catheter. (b) Laser balloon catheter. (c) High-intensity focused ultrasound (HIFU).*

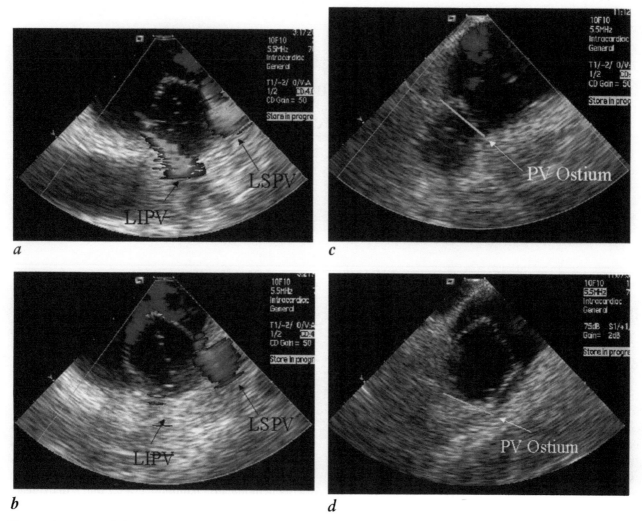

Figure 13.2 *Most balloon systems achieve better lesions when complete occlusion of the pulmonary vein (PV) is obtained. Intracardiac echocardiography is helpful in assessing balloon contact and position along the pulmonary vein. (a) Doppler flow through both the left inferior pulmonary vein (LIPV) and left superior pulmonary vein (LSPV). Note that the balloon has not been optimally deployed in the LIPV, as documented by the presence of blood flow between the PV ostium and the balloon, suggesting partial occlusion. (b) The balloon has been correctly deployed at the level of the ostia of the LIPV. Note that the flow of blood has been occluded, as evidenced by Doppler. (c) The balloon has been placed too far distal into the lumen of the right inferior pulmonary vein (RIPV). (d) Note the correct deployment of the balloon at the level of the antrum. (Courtesy of Drs Natale and Themistoclakis).*

circumvent this limitation, since the circumferential contact may be maximized and the negative thermal effects of ambient blood flow may be attenuated. ICE is useful in balloon placement and to verify contact.

The laser balloon uses photonic energy that causes volumetric heating of the tissue (Figure 13.2). By placing this balloon at a PV ostium, a periostial ring of laser energy may be projected onto the tissue, thus electrically isolating the PV. Furthermore, the optical fiber of this ablation catheter can also be utilized for reflectance spectroscopy. Consequently, continuous monitoring of the optical feedback differentiates contact with the atrial wall from when a portion of the catheter surface is "free floating" in the blood pool. The use of reflectance spectroscopy to provide real-time monitoring of the blanching effect of balloon–tissue contact optimizes lesion delivery.

High-intensity focused ultrasound (HIFU) balloons transmit ultrasonic energy in a ring pattern using gas or fluid as a reflector. The parabolic balloon focuses the ultrasound beam forward. The HIFU catheter is able to create lesions proximal to the lumen of the PVs, thus potentially reducing the likelihood of PV stenosis.

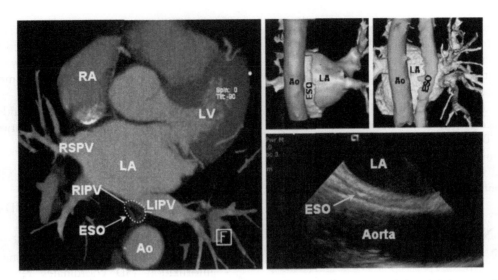

Figure 13.3 *During catheter ablation of atrial fibrillation, energy delivery to the posterior left atrium may result in damage to structures adjacent to the left atrium – including the esophagus and aorta. These structures exhibit marked variation in their location along the posterior left atrial wall. Real-time imaging of the esophagus and aorta can be performed using intracardiac echocardiographic imaging during the ablation procedure. Ao = aorta; ESO = esophagus; RA = right atrium; LA = left atrium; LV = left ventricle; RSPV = right superior pulmonary vein; RIPV = right inferior pulmonary vein; LIPV = left inferior pulmonary vein.*

Anatomic characteristics of the target sites such as ostial diameter larger than the balloon size, inability to reach the right inferior or other pulmonary vein ostia, ostial instability, early branching of the vein, and eccentric position of the ultrasound transducer in the vein, make it difficult to deliver energy effectively; however, attempts are being made to address many of these issues in newer balloon models.

These technologies face a number of challenges, including:

- Are the ablation sources safe?
- How much of the pulmonary venous antra can be ablated?
- Are the ablation lesions permanent?
- Given the inter-and intra-patient variability in PV size and morphology, can they be used in the majority of patients?

ARE THE ABLATION SOURCES SAFE?

Electrical isolation of the PVs can be accomplished by catheter ablation at or just proximal to the pulmonary vein–left atrium (PV–LA) junction. The technical complexity of the procedure, the possible formation of char and thrombosis secondary to the disruption of the endothelium by radiofrequency (RF) ablation, the risk of atria-esophageal fistula, and pulmonary venous stenosis when ablation is performed within the ostium represent some of the issues associated

with this procedure. These structures exhibit marked variation in their location along the posterior left atrial wall. In this respect, real-time imaging of the esophagus, the aorta, and the PVs can be performed using intracardiac echocardiographic imaging during the ablation procedure to potentially reduce the possibility of such complications (Figure 13.3).

Cryoablation technology has the potential to be a safer means of ablating cardiac tissue. Short-term complications include acute tissue hemorrhage, hemoptysis, and phrenic nerve paralysis. Three months after cryoablation of the PVs, canine cardiac tissue exhibited no collagen or cartilage formation. Furthermore, none of the animals had evidence of PV stenosis. The cure rate with cryoablation as the sole ablation tool is about 60–65%, with no evidence of PV stenosis.

Laser energy should not be applied through blood, since it is absorbed by blood. Therefore, lasing through blood reduces lesion size and increases the risk of thrombus formation. On the other hand, placing a balloon catheter in contact with the endocardium can provide a bloodless interface of balloon–tissue contact. Visualization of this balloon–tissue interface using an endoscopic fiber within the balloon, plus an adjustable location of energy delivery, can potentially allow PV isolation without thrombus. Pathologic examination revealed no PV stenosis when lesions were delivered outside the PVs, no pericardial damage, minor lung lesions without pleural perforation, minimal endothelial disruption, and, in the presence of adequate heparinization, no endocardial charring and overlying thrombus.

HIFU-mediated AF ablation has shown promising results. Since 2003, about 60 patients have been treated using this system. With improved catheter design, the success rate of AF ablation has increased from about 50% to 80%, without evidence of PV stenosis. Phrenic nerve paralysis remains a potential complication. The preliminary human study results need to be confirmed in larger series.

ASSESSMENT OF MORPHOLOGIC VARIANTS TO GUIDE ABLATION

The significant variability in the pulmonary venous morphology and orientation can be appreciated by pre-procedural magnetic resonance imaging (MRI) or computed tomography (CT) imaging (Figure 13.4). The top images in Figure 13.4 are MRI-based 3D surface renderings of the LA–PVs from two patients; note the contrast between the relatively "normal" 4 PVs anatomy (right) versus the distal coalescence of the left PVs into a large common

PV prior to joining the LA (left). The bottom images are internal endolumenal projections of the right-sided PVs. Note the difference between the two discreet PVs (left) versus the variable number of PVs (middle, right).

The workflow for performing image-guided therapy to aid catheter ablation of atrial fibrillation consists of 4 steps:

1. Acquisition of the high-definition MRI or CT angiograms.
2. Use of software tools to generate 3D constructs of the chamber(s) of interest.
3. Integrating/aligning this 3D CT/MR image with real-time electroanatomic mapping location information (3D coordinates represented by green dots), such that they are in an identical orientation.
4. Manipulation of the ablation catheter (blue-green icon) within the chamber in a real-time fashion (Figure 13.5).

Using a combination of external 3D surface reconstruction and internal projections, the integrated 3D CT/MR images can guide the real-time placement

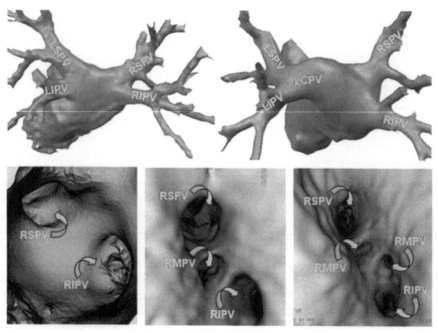

Figure 13.4 *The significant variability in the pulmonary venous morphology and orientation can be appreciated by pre-procedural MRI or CT imaging. The top images are MRI-based 3D surface renderings of the LA–PVs from two patients; note the contrast between the relatively "normal" 4 PVs anatomy (right) versus the distal coalescence of the left PVs into a large common PV prior to joining the LA (left). The bottom images are internal endolumenal projections of the right-sided PVs. Note the difference between the two discreet PVs (left) versus the variable number of middle PVs (middle, right). LIPV = left inferior pulmonary vein; LSPV = left superior pulmonary vein; RIPV = right inferior pulmonary vein; RSPV = right superior pulmonary vein; RMPV = right middle pulmonary vein; LCPV = left common pulmonary vein.*

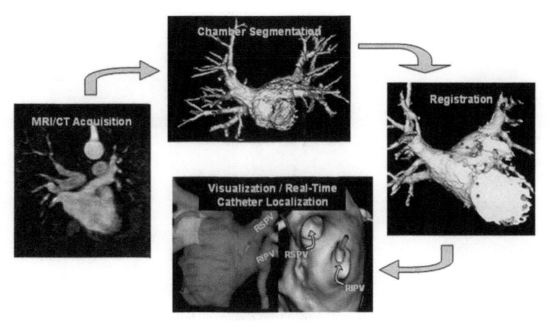

Figure 13.5 *The workflow for performing image-guided therapy to aid catheter ablation of atrial fibrillation consists of 4 steps: (1) acquisition of the high-definition MRI or CT angiograms; (2) use of software tools to generate 3D constructs of the chamber(s) of interest; (3) integrating/aligning this 3D CT/MR image with real-time electroanatomic mapping location information (3D coordinates represented by green dots), such that they are in an identical orientation; and (4) manipulation of the ablation catheter (blue-green icon) within the chamber in a real-time fashion. RSPV = right superior pulmonary vein; RIPV = right inferior pulmonary vein.*

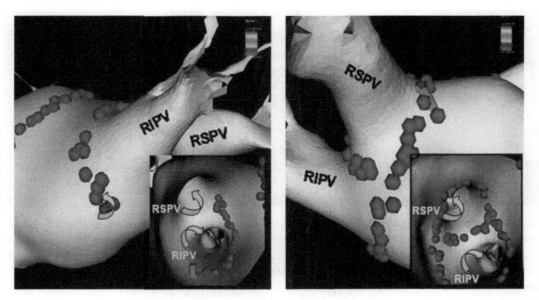

Figure 13.6 *Using a combination of external 3D surface rendered and internal projections, the integrated 3D CT/MR images can guide the real-time placement of catheter ablation lesions (red dots) to electrically isolate the pulmonary veins. RSPV = right superior pulmonary vein; RIPV = right inferior pulmonary vein.*

of catheter ablation lesions (red dots) to electrically isolate the pulmonary veins (Figure 13.6).

Looking at Figure 13.7, in addition to ablation points (red dots), other regions of interest can also be displayed on the 3D surface rendering (left image).

Because the 3D CT/MR images are pre-acquired images, a real-time electroanatomic map can also be generated and displayed in a separate window (right image) to provide further guide to mapping and ablation.

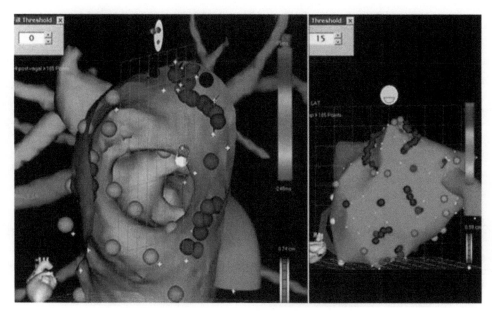

Figure 13.7 *In addition to ablation points (red dots), other regions of interest can also be displayed on the 3D surface rendering (left image). Because the 3D CT/MR images are pre-acquired images, a real-time electroanatomic map can also be generated and displayed in a separate window (right image) to provide a further guide to catheter mapping and ablation.*

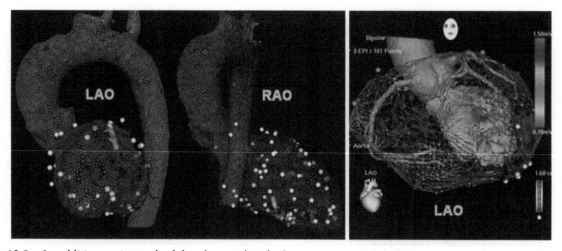

Figure 13.8 *In addition to its applicability for atrial arrhythmias, image-guided therapy can also be employed to guide catheter mapping and ablation of ventricular tachycardia. Left: a 3D CT rendering of the left ventricle and aorta are shown in this post-MI patient with scar-related ventricular tachycardia (VT) (the blue/white icon = mapping cathete). Right: in this patient with hypertrophic cardiomyopathy-related VT, a 3D CT rendering of the aortic root/coronaries (red) and LV endocardium (green) is shown registered to the epicardial electroanatomic map (wire frame mesh) to help guide catheter mapping and ablation. LAO = left anterior oblique; RAO = right anterior oblique.*

Besides its applicability for atrial arrhythmias, image-guided therapy can also be employed to guide catheter mapping and ablation of ventricular tachycardia. Looking at Figure 13.8 (left) a 3D CT

rendering of the left ventricle and aorta are shown in this post-MI patient with scar-related VT (the blue/white icon = mapping cathete). In this patient (right) with hypertrophic cardiomyopathy-related VT, a 3D

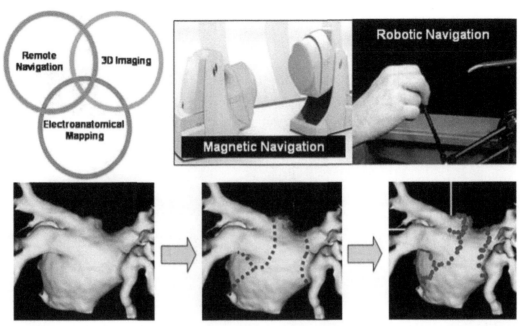

Figure 13.9   *The future of image-guided therapy will probably involve the integration of three technologies: 3D imaging (CT/MRI/ultrasound), electroanatomic mapping, and remote magnetic/robotic navigation. The eventual treatment paradigm may be: (1) obtain a 3D patient-specific image, (2) plan the ablation strategy, and (3) use a remote navigation methodology to navigate the ablation catheter to these locations (using electroanatomic mapping to provide real-time feedback as to catheter position).*

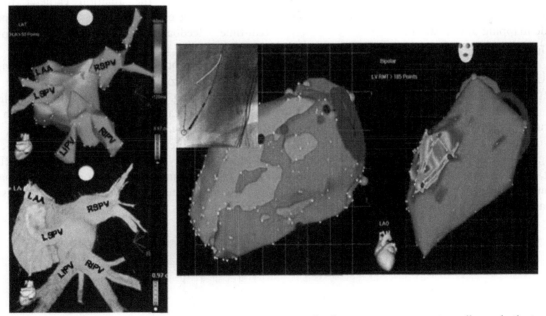

Figure 13.10   *The integration of magnetic remote navigation with electroanatomic mapping allows facile intracardiac mapping. Left: the porcine left atrium and pulmonary veins were remotely mapped using these technologies; note the similarity to the 3D CT rendering of the anatomy. Right: the porcine left ventricular endocardial surface was mapped using either standard manual (green shell) or remote magnetic (purple shells) manipulation; note both the similarity of chamber volumes (left) and the ability to perform sinus rhythm substrate mapping to identify the chronic anterior wall myocardial infarction. LAA = left atrial appendage; LIPV = left inferior pulmonary vein; LSPV = left superior pulmonary vein; RIPV = right inferior pulmonary vein; RSPV = right superior pulmonary vein.*

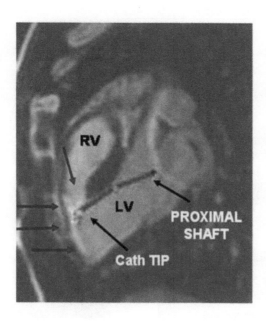 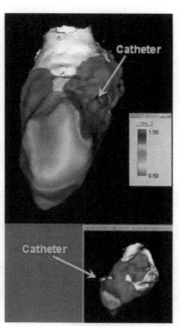

Figure 13.11 *Ultimately, real-time visualization of intracardiac catheters may be realized with MR imaging; i.e. interventional MRI (iMRI). Left: MR imaging of this porcine model of healed myocardial infarction reveals the hyperenhanced anterior wall scar (blue arrows), to which an MRI-compatible mapping catheter was manipulated in a real-time fashion. Right: a left ventricular substrate map is generated by displaying sinus rhythm electrogram amplitude values onto a 3D rendering of the chamber. RV = right ventricle; LV = left ventricle.*

CT rendering of the aortic root/coronaries (red) and LV endocardium (green) is shown registered to the epicardial electroanatomic map (wire frame mesh) to help guide mapping and ablation.

THE FUTURE OF IMAGE-GUIDED THERAPY

The future of image-guided therapy will probably involve the integration of three technologies: 3D imaging (CT/MRI/ultrasound), electroanatomic mapping, and remote magnetic/robotic navigation. The eventual treatment paradigm may be: (1) obtain a 3D patient-specific image, (2) plan the ablation strategy, and (3) use a remote navigation methodology to navigate the ablation catheter to these locations (using electroanatomic mapping to provide real-time feedback as to catheter position) (Figures 13.9–13.11).

The integration of magnetic remote navigation with electroanatomic mapping allows facile intracardiac mapping. Ultimately, real-time visualization of intracardiac catheters may be realized with MRI; i.e., *interventional* MRI (*iMRI*). Similarly, there remains the potential for real-time 3D echocardiographic imaging. Nevertheless, at this time, 2D ICE is the best real-time imaging modality to accompany fluoroscopy for many interventional electrophysiology applications.

Index

Note: **Bold** type denotes figures

3-D echocardiography 133–44
    alcohol septal ablation in hypertrophic
        cardiomyopathy 141, **142**
    anatomy assessment, electrophysiology
        studies 138–40, **139–40**
    ASDs 140–1, **141**
    cardiac masses 141–2
    chamber volume and function 133–4,
        134
    congenital heart disease assessment
        140–1
    fossa ovalis **139**
    future applications 133–44, 149–51,
        152
    interatrial septum **139**, 139–40, **140**
    left ventricular dyssynchrony 134–6
    myocardial perfusion 134–6
    potential utilities 141–2
    pulmonary veins **140**
    regional wall motion abnormalities
        134–6, **135**
    TDI 136
    valve assessment 136–8, **136–8**
    VSDs 140–1, **141**
3-D endoscopic reconstruction,
        pulmonary veins **81–3**

ablation
    AF *see* atrial fibrillation ablation
    VT *see* ventricular tachycardia
        ablation
abnormal anatomy
    LAA 45–9
    left atrial structures 45–58
    PVs 49–58
abnormalities, regional wall motion
        134–6, **135**
adult congenital heart disease
        125, **128**
agitated saline contrast, PFO 118, **119**
alcohol septal ablation, hypertrophic
        cardiomyopathy 141, **142**
aliasing effect, Doppler
        echocardiography 7, **7**
Amplatzer
    ASDs 120, **121**
    PFO **118**, 118

anatomic definition, right atrium
        105–14
anatomic structure identification,
        atrial fibrillation ablation 62–7
anatomic variations
    atrial fibrillation ablation 67–9
    interatrial septum 35, **36**
    pulmonary veins 67–9
anatomy
    abnormal *see* abnormal anatomy
    ASDs 118–19, **119**
    assessment, electrophysiology studies
        138–40, **139–40**
    atrial chambers 11–13
    AVMs 121, **122**
    gross heart 11
    interatrial septum 12
    LAA 91–3
    left atrium 12–13
    left ventricular outflow tract
        disease 123
    PFO 115–16, **116**
    pulmonary vein stenosis 123
    pulmonary veins **60–1**
    right atrium 11–12
    VSDs 120
aneurysms, IAS 35–8, **100**
antrum isolation, circular mapping
        catheter **72–7**, 72–7
aorta, intracardiac phased-array
        echocardiography imaging 15, **18**
aortic stenosis (AS) 123–5, **126–7**
ASDs *see* atrial septal defects
assessment
    anatomy, electrophysiology studies
        138–40, **139–40**
    chamber volume and function
        133–4, **134**
    congenital heart disease 140–1
    left ventricular dyssynchrony 134–6
    myocardial perfusion 134–6
    regional wall motion abnormalities
        134–6, **135**
    valve **136–8**, 136–8
atrial chambers
    gross anatomy 11–13
    home view 13–14, **14**, 17

imaging modalities 13
intracardiac phased-array
    echocardiography imaging 13–30
key points 17
atrial fibrillation
    LAA 47–8, 50
    LAA transcatheter occlusion 91–8
    pulmonary veins 53, **54–7**
atrial fibrillation ablation 59–89
    anatomic structure identification
        62–7
    anatomic variations 67–9
    antrum isolation **72–7**, 72–7
    balloon catheters 145–7
    catheter contact 77–86, 145–7, **146**
    circular mapping catheter 69–77,
        69–85
    complications, early detection 86–8,
        87–8
    cryoablation balloon catheter 145–7
    damage **147**
    Doppler flow recordings 81, **86**
    esophagus 66–7, **66–7**
    HIFU 145–7
    ICE recordings 69–70, 73–5
    LAA **62**
    laser balloon catheter 145–7
    left atrium **63**
    microbubbles 9, 81–6, **85–8**
    morphologic variants 148–52,
        148–52
    pulmonary artery **65**
    pulmonary veins 59–68, **60–1**, 63–8
    safety, ablation sources 147–8
    SVC-RA junction 65, **65**
    titrating energy delivery 77–86
    transseptal puncture 61–2, **61–2**
atrial flutter
    cavotricuspid isthmus 107–9
    LAA 48–9, 50
atrial septal defects (ASDs) 118–20,
        119–21
    3-D echocardiography 140–1, **141**
    Amplatzer 120, **121**
    anatomy 118–19, **119**
    Helex 120, **120**
    Sideris transcatheter patch **121**

atrioventricular nodal re-entry
    tachycardia (AVNRT)
  ablation **111**
  right atrium 109
AVMs *see* pulmonary arteriovenous
    malformations
AVNRT *see* atrioventricular nodal
    re-entry tachycardia

balloon catheters 145, 145–7, **146**
  cryoablation 145–7
  HIFU 145–7
  laser 145–7
basics
  echocardiographic imaging 3–4, **4**
  sonography 3–8, **3–8**

cardiac masses, 3-D echocardiography
    141–2
CardioSEAL, PFO 116–18, **117**
catheter ablation, atrial fibrillation
    see atrial fibrillation ablation
catheter contact, atrial fibrillation
    ablation 77–86, 145–7, **146**
cavotricuspid isthmus
  ablation, post **112**
  atrial flutter 107–9
  intracardiac phased-array
    echocardiography imaging 14, **16**
  phased-array image **111**, **112**
  progressive isthmus swelling **112**
  right atrium 107–9
  variation **110**
chamber volume and function,
    assessment 133–4, **134**
circular mapping catheter
  antrum isolation 72–7, **72–7**
  atrial fibrillation ablation 69–77, **69–85**
  pulmonary veins, 3-D endoscopic
    reconstruction **81–3**
color Doppler echocardiography 7–8, **8**
  interatrial septum **19**
  PFO 116–18, **117**
  pulmonary veins 21, 22, 23, 52, 63, **64**
common ostium, pulmonary veins
    67–8, **67–8**
complications, early detection, atrial
    fibrillation ablation 86–8, **87–8**
congenital catheterization laboratory
    115–28
  adult congenital heart disease 125, **128**
  AS 123–5, **126–7**
  ASDs 118–20, **119–21**
  AVMs 121, **122**
  left ventricular outflow tract disease
    123–5, **126–7**
  PFO 115–18
  pulmonary vein stenosis 123, **124–5**
  TOF 125, **128**
  VSDs 120–1, **122**

congenital heart disease
  3-D echocardiography 140–1
  assessment 140–1
continuous wave Doppler 7, **7**
contraindications, ICE 8–9
coronary sinus (CS)
  IPE **131**
  ostium, right atrium 109
  short-axis view, intracardiac
    phased-array echocardiography
    imaging **16**
crista terminalis
  intracardiac phased-array
    echocardiography imaging 13–17,
    14, **15**
  mechanical transducer images **108**
  right atrium 107, **107**
cryoablation balloon catheter 145, 145–7

damage, atrial fibrillation ablation 147
developments
  historical 1
  ICE systems 1–3
Doppler flow mapping, trade-offs 8, **8**
Doppler flow patterns
  LAA 45–6, 50
  pulmonary veins 50–3
Doppler flow recordings, atrial
    fibrillation ablation 81, **86**
Doppler shift principles 6, **6–7**
  aliasing effect 7, **7**
  color Doppler echocardiography
    7–8, **8**
  continuous wave Doppler 7, **7**
  Doppler flow mapping 8, **8**
  pulsed-wave Doppler 7–8, **8**

echocardiographic imaging, basics
    3–4, **4**
electroanatomic mapping **151**, **152**
esophagus, atrial fibrillation ablation
    66–7, **66–7**
eustachian ridge, intracardiac
    phased-array echocardiography
    imaging 14, **16**

fossa ovalis
  3-D echocardiography **139**
  intracardiac phased-array
    echocardiography imaging **19**, **20**
  right atrium 109–10
future applications, 3-D
    echocardiography 133–44,
    149–51, **152**
future, image-guided therapies 145–52,
    149–51

Helex, ASDs 120, **120**
high-intensity focused ultrasound (HIFU)
    balloons 145, 145–7

historical developments 1
home view, atrial chambers 13–14, **14**, 17
hypertrophic cardiomyopathy, alcohol
    septal ablation 141, **142**

IAS *see* interatrial septum
IASA *see* interatrial septal aneurysm
ICE systems 1–3
  mechanical/rotational transducers
    1–3, **2**
  phased-array transducers 1–3, **2**, **3**
imaging modalities, atrial chambers 13
indications, ICE 8–9
interatrial septal aneurysm (IASA) **100**
  PFO 35–8
interatrial septum (IAS) 31–8
  3-D echocardiography **139**, 139–40,
    140
  abnormalities 35, **36**
  anatomic variations 35, **36**
  anatomy 12
  aneurysms 35–8, **100**
  catheterization 99–103
  development 31, **32–3**
  double septum **100**
  imaging techniques 31–5, **33–5**
  intracardiac phased-array
    echocardiography imaging
    14–17, **16**, **19**, **20**
  left atrial catheterization 99–103
  lipomatous hypertrophy **36**
  PFO 35–8
  TEE 31
  tenting 99–102, **100**, **101**, **112**
  thick **100**
  transseptal catheterization 99–103
intrapericardial echocardiography (IPE)
    129–31, **129–31**

Koch triangle 12, 106, 109

LAA *see* left atrial appendage
LAD *see* left anterior descending
    coronary artery
laser balloon catheter 145, 145–7
left anterior descending coronary
    artery (LAD), IPE **130**
left atrial appendage (LAA)
  abnormal anatomy 45–9
  anatomy 91–3
  assessment 45–9
  atrial fibrillation 47–8, 50
  atrial fibrillation ablation 62
  atrial flutter 48–9, **50**
  Doppler flow patterns 45–6, 50
  function 91–3
  ICE 45, **49**
  ICE role, LAA occlusion 94–7
  intracardiac phased-array
    echocardiography imaging **19**

IPE 131
occluder devices 93, 93–4
occlusion 91–8
pathologic specimens 92
PLAATO device 93, 93–4
SEC 45, **46**, **49**
sinus rhythm 46–7, 50
TEE 45, **47**, **48**
TEE role, LAA occlusion 94–7
thrombus development **113**
transcatheter occlusion 91–8
TTE 45, **48**
visualisation 94
Watchman device **93**, 93–4
left atrial structures, abnormal anatomy 45–58
left atrium
    anatomy 12–13
    atrial fibrillation ablation 63
    false tendon **68**
    intracardiac phased-array
        echocardiography imaging
        13–17, **16**
    MRI view **59**
    thrombus development **113**
    transseptal catheterization 99–103
left pulmonary veins see pulmonary
        veins
left sinus of Valsalva, VT **43**
left ventricle, normal **41**
left ventricular dyssynchrony
    3-D echocardiography 134–6
    assessment 134–6
left ventricular outflow tract disease
    123–5, **126–7**
    anatomy 123
    AS 123–5
left ventricular procedures, VT ablation
    39–42, 41–4
limitations, ICE 9

M-mode echocardiographic imaging
    5–6, **6**
magnetic/robotic remote navigation
    151, **152**
mapping catheter, circular see circular
    mapping catheter
mechanical/rotational transducers, ICE
    systems 1–3, **2**
microbubbles, atrial fibrillation ablation
    9, 81–6, **85–8**
mitral regurgitation (MR) **136–8**, 136–8
morphologic variants, atrial fibrillation
    ablation **148–52**, 148–52
motion abnormalities, regional wall
    134–6, **135**
MR see mitral regurgitation
myocardial perfusion
    3-D echocardiography 134–6
    assessment 134–6

PA see pulmonary artery
parallel processing, vs serial
        processing 5–6, **6**
patent foramen ovale (PFO) 115–18
    agitated saline contrast 118, **119**
    Amplatzer **118**, 118
    anatomy 115–16, **116**
    CardioSEAL 116–18, **117**
    color Doppler echocardiography
        116–18, **117**
    interatrial septum 35–8
pectinate muscles, intracardiac
        phased-array echocardiography
        imaging 13–17, **15**
pericardial echocardiography
    see intrapericardial
    echocardiography
PFO see patent foramen ovale
phased-array transducers,
        ICE systems 1–3, **2**, **3**, 4–5, **5**
piezoelectric crystal transducers 3, 3–5
PLAATO device, LAA **93**, 93–4
pulmonary arteriovenous malformations
    (AVMs) 121, **122**
    anatomy 121, **122**
pulmonary artery (PA)
    atrial fibrillation ablation 65
    normal **40**
pulmonary valve, normal **40**
pulmonary vein isolation (PVI) 53, **54–7**
pulmonary vein stenosis 123, **124–5**
    anatomy 123
    radiofrequency ablation 123, **124**
    sinus venosus ASD repair 123, **124**
pulmonary veins (PVs)
    3-D echocardiography **140**
    3-D endoscopic reconstruction **81–3**
    abnormal anatomy 49–58
    anatomic variations 67–9
    anatomy **60–1**
    assessment 49–57
    atrial fibrillation 53, **54–7**
    atrial fibrillation ablation 59–68,
        60–1, **63–8**
    color Doppler echocardiography 21,
        22, **23**, **52**, 63, **64**
    common ostium 67–8, **67–8**
    Doppler flow patterns 50–3
    false tendon **68**
    ICE 50, **52**
    intracardiac phased-array
        echocardiography imaging 21,
        22, **23**, 24–7
    long-axis view 21, **22**
    pulsed-wave Doppler **64**
    PVI 53, **54–7**
    sinus rhythm 53, **53**
    stenosis see pulmonary vein stenosis
    TEE 49, **51**, 53–6
    TTE 49–50, **54**

pulsed-wave Doppler 7–8, **8**
    pulmonary veins **64**
PVI see pulmonary vein isolation
PVs see pulmonary veins

radiofrequency catheter ablation,
        thrombus development **113**
RA–SVC junction, intracardiac
        phased-array echocardiography
        imaging 18
rationale, ICE 8–9
regional wall motion abnormalities,
        assessment 134–6, **135**
remote navigation 151, **152**
right atrial appendage, intracardiac
        phased-array echocardiography
        imaging 13–17, **15**
right atrium 105–14
    ablation catheter placement **109**
    anatomic definition 105–14
    anatomy 11–12
    AVNRT **109**
    cavotricuspid isthmus 107–9
    complex congenital heart disease 110
    coronary sinus ostium **109**
    crista terminalis 107, **107**
    fossa ovalis 109–10
    intracardiac phased-array
        echocardiography imaging 13–17,
        14, **15**, **16**
    intraprocedural monitoring 110–13
    mechanical transducer images
        106, **108**
    phased-array baseline image **106**
    sinoatrial node region **107**
    tachycardia 107–9
    transseptal puncture 109–10
right atrium–superior vena cava
        junction, intracardiac phased-
        array echocardiography imaging **18**
right pulmonary veins see pulmonary veins
right ventricle
    intracardiac phased-array
        echocardiography imaging 13–17,
        14, **16**
    normal **40**
right ventricle outflow tract, intracardiac
        phased-array echocardiography
        imaging **18**
right ventricular outflow tract (RVOT),
        normal **40**
right ventricular procedures, VT ablation
        39, **40–1**
RVOT see right ventricular outflow tract

safety, ablation sources 147–8
scan-line processing 5, **5**
SEC see spontaneous echo contrast
septal myectomy, hypertrophic
        cardiomyopathy 141, **142**

serial processing, vs parallel processing 5–6, **6**
Sideris double balloon patch, VSDs 120–1, **121–2**
Sideris transcatheter patch, ASDs **121**
sinoatrial node region, right atrium 107
sinus rhythm
  LAA 46–7, **50**
  pulmonary veins 53, **53**
sinus venosus ASD repair, pulmonary vein stenosis 123, **124**
Snell's law 3–4, **4**
sonography
  basics 3–8, **3–8**
  Snell's law 3–4, **4**
spontaneous echo contrast (SEC), LAA 45, 46, **49**
superior vena cava–right atrial (SVC–RA) junction, atrial fibrillation ablation 65, **65**
supravalvar aortic stenosis (AS) 123–5, **127**
SVC–RA junction *see* superior vena cava–right atrial junction
systems, ICE *see* ICE systems

TDI *see* Tissue Doppler imaging
TEE *see* transesophageal echocardiography

tetralogy of Fallot (TOF) 125, **128**
three-dimensional echocardiography *see* 3-D echocardiography
three-dimensional endoscopic reconstruction *see* 3-D endoscopic reconstruction
thrombus development, radiofrequency catheter ablation **113**
Tissue Doppler imaging (TDI), 3-D echocardiography 136
TOF *see* tetralogy of Fallot
transcatheter occlusion, LAA 91–8
transesophageal echocardiography (TEE)
  interatrial septum 31
  LAA 45, 47, **48**
  LAA occlusion 94–7
  pulmonary veins 49, **51**, 53–6
transseptal catheterization 99–103
transseptal puncture
  atrial fibrillation ablation 61–2, **61–2**
  intracardiac phased-array echocardiography imaging **20**
  right atrium 109–10
transthoracic echocardiography (TTE)
  LAA 45, **48**
  pulmonary veins 49–50, **54**
triangle of Koch 12, 106, 109

tricuspid valve, intracardiac phased-array echocardiography imaging 13–17, **14**, **16**
TTE *see* transthoracic echocardiography

valves
  assessment, 3-D echocardiography 136–8, **136–8**
  PV, normal **40**
  tricuspid valve, intracardiac phased-array echocardiography imaging 13–17, **14**, **16**
ventricular septal defects (VSDs) 120–1, **122**
  3-D echocardiography 140–1, **141**
  anatomy 120
  paramembranous 120–1, **122**
  Sideris double balloon patch 120–1, **121–2**
ventricular tachycardia (VT) ablation 39–44, **150**
  AVNRT **111**
  left sinus of Valsalva **43**
  left ventricular procedures 39–42, **41–4**
  other applications 42–4
  right ventricular procedures 39, **40–1**
VSDs *see* ventricular septal defects

Watchman device
  LAA **93**, 93–4

9781842143100